Advances in Drug Research

Volume 9

Advances in Drug Research

Series Editors

N. J. HARPER

*Sterling Winthrop, Research and Development
Newcastle upon Tyne, England*

and

ALMA B. SIMMONDS

*Chelsea College
University of London, England*

Volume 9

edited by Alma B. Simmonds

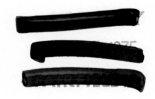

1974

ACADEMIC PRESS
LONDON NEW YORK SAN FRANCISCO
A Subsidiary of Harcourt Brace Jovanovich, Publishers

ACADEMIC PRESS INC. (LONDON) LTD
24–28 Oval Road
London NW1

US edition published by
ACADEMIC PRESS INC.
111 Fifth Avenue,
New York, New York 10003

Library of Congress Catalog Card Number: 64-24672
ISBN: 0-12-013309-1

PRINTED IN GREAT BRITAIN BY
WILLIAM CLOWES & SONS LIMITED
LONDON, BECCLES AND COLCHESTER

Contributors to Volume 9

R. HOWE, BSc, PhD, FRIC
Imperial Chemical Industries Ltd, Pharmaceuticals Division, Mereside, Alderley Park, Macclesfield, Cheshire, England

E. M. JEPSON, MD, FRCP
Central Middlesex Hospital, London, England

D. KRITCHEVSKY, BS, MS, PhD
The Wistar Institute of Anatomy and Biology, Thirty-sixth Street at Spruce, Philadelphia, Pennsylvania, USA

J. R. PARRATT, BPharm, MSc, PhD, FPS
Department of Physiology and Pharmacology, Royal College, University of Strathclyde, George Street, Glasgow, Scotland

E. M. VAUGHAN WILLIAMS, DM, DSc
Department of Pharmacology, University of Oxford, South Parks Road, Oxford, England

K. W. WALTON, MD, PhD, MRCS, FRCPath
Department of Experimental Pathology, The Medical School, University of Birmingham, England

Preface

"Advances in Drug Research", *Volume 9*, reviews the physiological, pharmacological and clinical aspects of ischaemic heart disease. The risk factors are many and there is a high mortality rate. The correlation of hyperlipidaemia with atherosclerosis and the resulting increased risk of coronary heart disease has long been known. Atherosclerosis of the coronary vessels may lead to coronary occlusions and infarction.

The research into hyperlipidaemia described in this volume is directed to the various plasma lipoproteins, their implications in atherogenesis and to the design of drugs which will correct abnormal lipoprotein patterns.

Many affected patients succumb to ventricular fibrillation. Research is described directed to effective antidysrhythmic drugs and to their proper utilization to save life. Coronary atherosclerosis may also contribute to imbalance between myocardial oxygen requirements and supply resulting in angina pectoris. A pharmacological basis for possible drug treatment completes this volume.

The interrelated contributions by a chemist, pharmacologists and clinicians illustrates the multidisciplinary nature of drug research.

I wish to express my thanks to the authors who lavished time and care on the preparation of their manuscripts and as always to Dorothy Sharp of Academic Press Inc. (London) Ltd for ensuring the high standard of book production.

July 1974

ALMA B. SIMMONDS

Contents

The Prevention of Ischaemic Heart Disease—Clinical Management[1]

E. M. JEPSON, MD, FRCP

Central Middlesex Hospital, London, England

It is exceptionally difficult to give advice on the prevention of a disease when one cannot be certain if it is present or not. Ischaemic heart disease begins to develop well before symptoms can be detected, and the interval between the first pathological changes and the appearance of clinical symptoms may be years. At present a management programme aimed at preventing ischaemic heart disease can only be based on hope. Nevertheless, it should at least be considered since ischaemic heart disease is the cause of death in about one third of men in the United Kingdom between the ages of 35 and 64 years. Although the figure for women is less than one in seven, the incidence is rising steadily.

1 Risk factors

In order to carry out a programme to prevent the disease, it is necessary to select at least those who are at the greatest risk. To detect these there are a few clues. Heredity is one of the factors but many patients with a family history of ischaemic heart disease have no detectable abnormality. If such an abnormality is found then genetic counselling of the parents before they embark on a family is a means of reducing the incidence in the population. Unalterable risk factors are blood group A, age and sex. The risk of ischaemic heart disease in women is increased by ovariectomy which suggests that the sex hormones are somehow involved. Also the oestrogen in oral contraceptives increases the risk of thrombotic episodes

---

[1] A talk given at the Society for Drug Research Symposium on Ischaemic Heart Disease, 26–27 September 1973.

(as compared with non-pregnant women) and may lead to myocardial infarction. Whether the oestrogen is a risk factor for all women, or only those with some other (probably hereditary) factor, is unknown, but the latter does seem probable. The occupation may also be a hazard. The general practitioner is at greater risk than the hospital consultant and, although this is well known in the medical profession, the current trend is away from hospital into general practice. Inevitably a shortage of men to run the bus transport in London has resulted in the appearance of buses manned by one man who of necessity is both driver and conductor —this combined function is unlikely to reduce the greater risk to drivers as compared with conductors. Social class has an influence, classes 4 and 5 being at greater risk than classes 1 and 2. A change in social class may be a risk in more ways than one.

The commonest habit which is a definite risk is smoking. The incidence of ischaemic heart disease is on average twice as high in those who smoke as those who do not. The number of cigarettes smoked per day and the age of starting to smoke are determining factors. There is some comfort for those smoking today for if they stop now, in approximately ten years' time their risk falls to the same as those who have never smoked. The heavy drinker of alcohol not only has a high incidence of ischaemic heart disease: he may also have detectable abnormalities in the blood lipids. The only safe beverage appears to be water, hard water being better than soft.

Diet has been implicated in many epidemiological studies related to ischaemic heart disease and people living on a sophisticated diet rich in saturated fat and refined sugar in the so-called developed countries are at much greater risk than those in the more rural or so-called backward areas. Gluttony and obesity are not by themselves risk factors, but coupled with other bad habits they can contribute to the development of the disease. Regular exercise is of great importance in the prevention of ischaemic heart disease and those who are entirely sedentary are at much greater risk. It might be possible to change the personality but it is very hard to change a man at high risk from a worrying hard-working and constantly twitching high-pressure business executive to one who is more suited to the cultivation of cabbages.

2 Hidden disease

Certain diseases which may not be detected by symptoms of their own and which may become manifest by ischaemic heart disease can be counted as risk factors. One of these is hypertension which is high on the list of dangerous disorders. Unknown elevation of blood pressure may first of all be discovered when ischaemic heart disease is the presenting symptom and, therefore, the simple recording of blood pressure is a vital part of a screening examination that a practitioner may carry out.

More difficult to discover is the presence of hyperlipidaemia which is a potent risk factor (see "Hyperlipidaemia" by K. W. Walton, p. 55). This may be primary or secondary to several disorders. As well as the excessive intake of alcohol, hidden thyroid insufficiency, chronic renal disease and pancreatic disorders can all lead to secondary hyperlipidaemia. Primary hyperlipidaemia may have no specific clinical signs but in many cases xanthomata are present or a corneal arcus is found.

Diabetes is commonly associated with ischaemic heart disease. In the detection of diabetes it is not sufficient to examine urine for glucose, it is necessary to examine the blood glucose after a high carbohydrate meal. Gout is also associated with ischaemic heart disease. A raised level of uric acid does not always lead to gout, but it may be one of the chemical abnormalities which predispose to the development of ischaemic heart disease.

Age (about which nothing can be done), high blood pressure and a raised plasma cholesterol are the best indicators of the risk in a particular individual of developing ischaemic heart disease.

3 Primary prevention

Having discussed the known risk factors we move on to management, the effects of which so far have been little more than minimal. The management before the symptoms of ischaemic heart disease have appeared is known as primary prevention, but this may be decades after the ischaemic heart disease began. Most trials and studies in primary prevention are based on dietary management in an attempt to lower the blood lipids which were not necessarily abnormal to start with. The unsaturated fat diet studied in Finland (Turpeinen, 1970) on otherwise normal (or seemingly normal) people over a period of six years seems to have been successful and possibly the prudent diet of the anticoronary club of New York (Christakis *et al.*, 1966) may also be successful although their results are hardly capable of being analysed statistically. A better conducted trial is now being carried out by the World Health Organization centred on Edinburgh, Prague, and Budapest (Oliver, 1970). In this trial clofibrate is being given to assess its value as a hypolipidaemic agent and the effect on the incidence of ischaemic heart disease.

4 Secondary prevention

Secondary prevention after a coronary thrombosis or myocardial infarct has occurred is even more difficult to evaluate. It seems that the risk factors which may have been present before the event no longer apply. Thus, high blood pressure and raised cholesterol levels have little influence on the subsequent course of events.

A diet with low saturated fat and cholesterol supplemented with polyunsaturated fats is most commonly used. Using such diets some improvements have been reported (Leven, 1966; Dayton et al., 1969). In this country the Medical Research Council trial showed no benefit at all to the patient (Medical Research Council, 1969). Certain drugs are under investigation in secondary prevention. Some results are available from the United States Coronary Drug Project (American Medical Association, 1972). The use of oestrogen led to a deterioration in those treated as did the dextro-isomer of thyroxine. Clofibrate is probably beneficial but still under trial. The trial of clofibrate carried out in Scotland and North East England (Dewar and Oliver, 1971) produced some results which were not those they expected to find. Patients with angina, or those who developed it after a myocardial infarct, did better on clofibrate than those without angina. The effect on the blood lipids did not affect the findings. The trial was designed to study one factor and revealed others of equal importance. It is certainly not the end of the tale.

Considering the treatment of an individual apart from a clinical trial, the management of hyperlipidaemia is the most interesting modern development. This depends on typing the lipid abnormality in the plasma. The division of hyperlipoproteinaemia into five types by Fredrickson et al. (1967) and the principal modes of treatment are shown in Table 1. It is mandatory in the first instance to attempt dietary management—it is less hazardous and far less costly than drug treatment. Certain types of hyperlipidaemia may require additional drug therapy. Of the three drugs in common use, cholestyramine is not a very easy powder to take and nicotinic acid has unpleasant side effects. Clofibrate is generally uncomplicated but expensive.

The management of hypertension is along standard lines by correction of the raised blood pressure. The treatment of patients with diabetes, some without recognizable symptoms, is now being studied in Bedford. Whether the correction by diet or sulphonylurea of an underlying defect of glucose metabolism will reduce or even increase the risk of ischaemic heart disease in these persons will not be known for many years. Efforts to correct hyperuricaemia with allopurinol are being made

TABLE 1

Clinical management of hyperlipoproteinaemia

Type[a]	Main lipoprotein constituent	Main lipid	Treatment
I	Chylomicrons	Triglyceride	Low fat diet, medium chain triglyceride
II	β-Lipoproteins	Cholesterol	Low saturated fat, low cholesterol and high unsaturated fat diet. Cholestyramine. Nicotinic acid
III	Intermediate (floating) β-lipoprotein	Cholesterol	Clofibrate
IV	Pre-β-lipoprotein	Triglyceride	Low calorie, low carbohydrate diet. Clofibrate. Nicotinic acid
V	Pre-β-lipoprotein and chylomicrons	Triglyceride	Low carbohydrate, low fat diet. Clofibrate. Nicotinic acid

[a] Fredrickson *et al.* (1967). See also "Hypolipidaemic Agents" by R. Howe on page 7.

but the effect on the risk of ischaemic heart disease is not yet known.

A management programme can be devised for the prevention of ischaemic heart disease once the chief risk factors have been identified, but we do not yet know for certain whether these measures are beneficial or not. There are indications that these measures are beneficial. Provided no additional harm is done to the patient, and in view of the fact that concrete results of trials will not be produced for many years to come, clinical management programmes for the prevention of ischaemic heart disease are justified.

References

American Medical Association (1972). *J. Amer. Med. Ass.* **220**, 996.

Christakis, G., Rinzlar, S. H., Archer, M., Winslow, G., Jampel, S., Stephenson, J., Friedman, G., Fein, H., Kraus, A. and Hamas, G. (1966). *Amer. J. Publ. Hlth.*, **56**, 299.

Dayton, S., Pearce, M. L., Hashimoto, S. D., Dixon, W. J. and Tomoyasu, W. (1969). *Circulation*, **40**, Sept. 11.

Dewar, H. A. and Oliver, M. F. (1971). *Brit. Med. J.* **iv**, 784.

Fredrickson, D. S., Levy, R. I. and Lees, R. S. (1967). *New England J. Med.* **276**, 94, 148, 215 and 273.

Leven, P. (1966). *Acta Med. Scand. Suppl.* **466**.
Oliver, M. F. (1970). *In* "Atherosclerosis" (Ed. R. J. Jones), p. 582. Springer Verlag, New York.
Turpeinen, O. (1970). *In* "Atherosclerosis" (Ed. R. J. Jones), p. 572. Springer Verlag, New York.

Hypolipidaemic Agents[1]

R. HOWE, BSc, PhD, FRIC

Imperial Chemical Industries Ltd., Pharmaceuticals Division, Mereside, Alderley Park, Macclesfield, Cheshire, England

1 Introduction

It is now widely accepted that there is a causal relationship between elevated plasma lipid levels and the development of atherosclerotic disease, which in turn leads to an increased coronary heart disease risk. Thus, it is considered therapeutically desirable to lower lipid levels to within the normal range by diet or by drugs. Proof that correction of lipid levels will automatically reduce the risk of coronary heart disease is still being sought.

Agents which illustrate the ways in which interference with biochemical processes may contribute to an observed reduction in lipid levels in mammals are reviewed here. It is not the purpose of the review to

[1] An expanded version of a talk given at the symposium "Perspectives in Ischaemic Heart Disease", Society for Drug Research, London, September 26–27, 1973.

present an exhaustive list of the many chemicals which have been claimed to lower lipid levels, or to discuss chemical synthesis. However, short sections describing plasma lipids and the classification of hyper-lipoproteinaemias are included to give perspective to subsequent discussion on the mode of action of hypolipidaemic agents.

2 Plasma lipids

In chemical terms there are four primary types of plasma lipids to consider: cholesterol, phospholipids, triglycerides, and free fatty acids. Free fatty acids travel in the blood bound to albumin and although at any given time their contribution to the total lipid level is low, their turnover is high. In quantitative terms the movement of free fatty acids and triglycerides are the major fat transport tasks that the blood carries out. Cholesterol and triglycerides are not present in the free form in blood, but are bound to special proteins and to other classes of blood lipid. The total packages are called lipoproteins, and four types are discussed below. The proteins impart solubility to the otherwise insol-uble lipids. Part of the cholesterol is esterified with long-chain fatty acids. Cholesterol and its esters and phospholipids, which constitute about two-thirds of the plasma lipid, have a much slower turnover rate than fatty acids. Most of the cholesterol in the blood is not there as cargo for delivery to tissues, but as a structural component of lipoproteins, some of which can be looked upon as vehicles for transport of other lipids, particularly triglycerides. Triglycerides are transported to tissues which use them as an energy source or store them. They may be of immediate dietary origin or may have been synthesized in the liver.

Two basic types of lipoproteins are designated α or high density and β or low density according to their behaviour on electrophoresis and preparative ultracentrifugation. These differ not only in the proportions of cholesterol and phospholipid which they contain, but also in the amount and nature of their protein components. The species known as pre-β-lipoproteins or very low density lipoproteins are composed of α- and β-lipoproteins and triglycerides of hepatic origin. If the α- and β-lipoproteins are considered as vehicles for triglyceride transport, then the pre-β-lipoprotein is the loaded vehicle, and naturally the load of tri-glyceride may vary. The liver secretes nascent pre-β-lipoproteins which become pre-β-lipoproteins by transfer of polypeptides from α-lipopro-teins. Triglycerides of dietary origin are transported in the form of chylo-microns, the largest lipoproteins. These are large neutral fat particles which contain only small amounts of protein and very much less choles-terol and phospholipid than the other lipoproteins. They are formed in intestinal cells during fat absorption, and their triglyceride components appear to turn over rather faster than those of pre-β-lipoproteins.

Table 1 gives the relative sizes of the lipoproteins and representative values for the proportions of their constituents. Structurally, lipoproteins are thought to consist of a hydrophobic core of triglycerides and cholesterol esters surrounded by a thin hydrophilic coat of phospholipid, free cholesterol and protein. Serum lipoproteins have been reviewed by Scanu and Wisdom (1972) and by Hamilton (1972).

TABLE 1

Lipoprotein, proportion of constituents, by weight

	α-Lipoprotein (0·01 μm)	β-Lipoprotein (0·02 μm)	Pre-β-lipoprotein (0·03–0·09 μm)	Chylomicron (0·1–0·4 μm)
Protein	52	21	10	1
Triglycerides	8	9	55	90
Total cholesterol	18	47	16	4
Phospholipid	22	23	19	5

3 Hyperlipoproteinaemia

Hyperlipidaemia was equated initially with high serum cholesterol levels, but Carlson (1960) recognized the high incidence of elevated plasma triglyceride levels in patients with clinical manifestations of atherosclerosis such as coronary artery disease. The more recent realization that plasma lipids are transported in the form of lipoproteins requires that hyperlipidaemia should be interpreted in terms of the nature of the hyperlipoproteinaemia rather than in terms of hypercholesterolaemia or hypertriglyceridaemia. It may be that the chylomicron level is high, or the β-lipoprotein level, or the pre-β-lipoprotein level, or combinations of these covering a spectrum of possibilities. Fredrickson *et al.* (1967) simplified the picture by recognizing five main types of hyperlipoproteinaemic conditions, a classification which has recently been modified slightly by the Beaumont Committee of the World Health Organization (Beaumont *et al.*, 1970). Type I is high in chylomicrons, type IIa high in β-lipoproteins, type IIb high in β- and pre-β-lipoproteins, type III high in intermediate β-lipoproteins of abnormally low density, type IV high in pre-β-lipoproteins, and type V high in pre-β-lipoproteins and chylomicrons. Looked at in another way, types IIa and IIb are characterized roughly by very high cholesterol levels, and types I, IV, and V by very high triglyceride levels. Serum lipoproteins must be considered as potential atherogenic agents, since their properties determine whether they can invade the arterial wall and deposit their lipid therein. β-Lipoprotein appears to be the principal transport vehicle for lipid permeating the arterial wall. It is selectively retained in the wall and deposits its lipid there (Walton and Williamson, 1968).

Little is known about the specific biochemical defects which lead to hyperlipoproteinaemias. Raised levels of chylomicrons are thought to occur because specific lipases necessary for their breakdown are deficient or absent (types I and V). Pre-β-lipoprotein levels may be high because of enhanced production by the liver in response to increased hepatic triglyceride synthesis, or because of decreased peripheral utilization (types IV, IIb, and V). β-Lipoproteins are thought to arise mainly by catabolic removal of triglycerides from pre-β-lipoprotein, but there may be some contribution from chylomicron catabolism. They may accumulate because of decreased removal by the liver, or as a consequence of increased production of pre-β-lipoprotein, leading to amounts of β-lipoprotein which exceed the normal degradative capacity (types IIa and IIb). Removal of all triglyceride-rich particles may be delayed if adipose and muscle cells are unresponsive (type V). A block in the normal conversion of pre-β- to β-lipoprotein results in accumulation of intermediate β-lipoprotein (type III) (Blohm, 1972; Levy and Rifkind, 1973).

Ideally, drug treatment should be related to the nature of the lipoprotein abnormality, and it would be naive to expect that one chemical could correct all abnormalities. A particular lipid abnormality may be due to a single biochemical defect and if that defect could be identified, then a specific agent could be sought to correct it. Lipid metabolism is extremely complex and involves many enzymic steps any of which could be defective. It is quite possible that two entirely separate defects could lead to final lipoprotein patterns sufficiently similar to be classified as a particular Fredrickson type (Lewis, 1973). Again, it should not be expected that a single chemical could correct both defects. Thus, a future aim should be to characterize a patient's biochemical defect and then treat it with a drug specific for that defect.

4   Hypolipidaemic agents

Although it is now recognized that the nature of lipoproteins and their serum levels are the important factors, the work described here has been directed mainly towards lowering cholesterol and triglyceride levels by whatever possible means. The mechanism has been sought later. This has been, and still is, an interesting but not wholly conclusive exercise because of the complex interrelationships which exist in lipid metabolism, and the links with carbohydrate metabolism. For example, a decrease in serum cholesterol level may be the result of reduced hepatic triglyceride synthesis. Less β-lipoprotein, of which cholesterol is the major component, would need to be synthesized to aid triglyceride transport from the liver. Further, work with relevant isolated enzyme systems may not always be meaningful if for metabolism, distribution, or transport reasons the compounds which affect those enzymes do not reach them efficiently *in vivo*. Use of non-physiological concentrations *in vitro* may provide results which have no bearing on effects observed *in vivo*. Compounds which act on several enzyme systems or which act *in vivo* by indirect mechanisms add to the difficulty of interpreting results. Species differences in lipid metabolism and transport and in the effect of drugs on those lipids make extrapolation from one species to another somewhat hazardous.

In the following section compounds which lower lipid levels in mammals and which affect a relevant enzyme system are discussed. It should be noted that partial inhibition of steps that are not rate-limiting may cause no net decrease in cholesterol or triglyceride biosynthesis. Many of the compounds, which are of diverse structures, affect more than one enzyme system and it is not possible to group them decisively by type of action or type of structure. To provide a thread of continuity, compounds are considered under five broad and overlapping headings in the following order: (1) compounds which inhibit endogenous synthesis of cholesterol; (2) compounds which stimulate catabolic removal of cholesterol; (3) compounds which lower triglyceride production; (4) compounds which stimulate removal of triglyceride; and (5) compounds which interfere with absorption or reabsorption of sterols or bile acids. When a compound is introduced as having a particular type of action, other possible actions are considered at the same time.

Many enzymic reactions are involved in cholesterol biosynthesis, but inhibition of some of them may not be beneficial. Some of the biosynthetic intermediates are shown in Fig. 1. Some intermediates, which will not be mentioned in the discussion, have been omitted.

Compounds which exert their effect on stages prior to β-hydroxy-β-methylglutaryl-CoA formation could interfere with metabolic reactions other than the biosynthesis of cholesterol, for example fatty acid biosynthesis, which is of prime interest in the context of lipid levels. A study of the separate incorporation of labelled acetate and labelled mevalonate into cholesterol in the presence of an inhibitor can discriminate between those compounds which exert a more or less general block on acetate metabolism and those which affect primarily the pathway

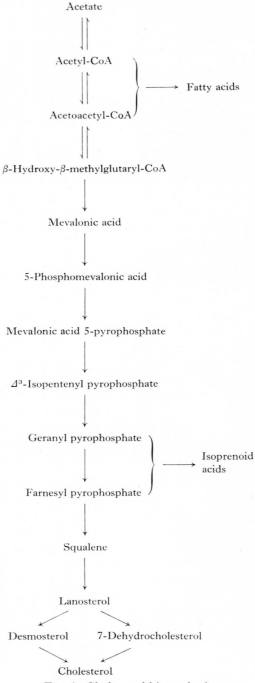

FIG. 1. Cholesterol biosynthesis.

reserved for cholesterol synthesis (Tavormina and Gibbs, 1957). Interruption of the sequence after squalene cyclization may result in the abnormal accumulation of steroidal precursors of cholesterol, and these may contribute to the development of atherosclerosis (Beher *et al.*, 1957). Except for being involved in the mammalian biosynthesis of coenzyme Q, which is a relatively minor pathway, mevalonic acid appears to be involved solely in the biosynthesis of sterols (Glorr and Wiss, 1959; Crombie, 1957). Moreover, a metabolic pathway exists for hepatic disposal of polyisoprenoid precursors of squalene (Popjak, 1959; Popjak *et al.*, 1960). Thus, it looks attractive to inhibit the biosynthetic steps between mevalonic acid and squalene. The area has been examined, but not yet thoroughly explored.

4.1 CHOLESTEROMIMETIC AGENTS

In experimental animals and in man, cholesterol biosynthesis is controlled by a negative feedback control system. Cholesterol-rich diets, which increase cholesterol in the plasma–liver pool, trigger an inhibition of the first irreversible step, the rate-limiting reduction of β-hydroxy-β-methylglutaryl-CoA to mevalonic acid (Bhattathiry and Siperstein, 1963). Efforts have been made to produce "cholesteromimetic" agents which could operate this negative feedback by an allosteric mechanism. A series of nitrogen isosteres of cholesterol-like compounds (1) to (8) was produced by Counsell *et al.* (1962a). 22,25-Diazacholestanol (1) decreased the incorporation of labelled acetate into cholesterol by rat liver homogenates, and it did so to a greater extent than it decreased the incorporation of labelled mevalonate (Ranney and Counsell, 1962). Incorporation of acetate into β-hydroxy-β-methylglutaryl-CoA was essentially unimpaired, whereas incorporation into mevalonate was reduced, implying inhibition of β-hydroxy-β-methylglutaryl-CoA reductase. In normal and hypercholesterolaemic rats the compound lowered cholesterol levels, apparently by the desired mechanism. Analogues (2) and (3) were not active in hypercholesterolaemic rats, (4) was active, and (5) and (6) progressively more potent as the nitrogen atom was moved towards the end of the side chain. Insertion of a second nitrogen into (6) at position 20 (compound 7) or position 22 (compound 8) lowered potency (Counsell *et al.*, 1962b; 1965). Alteration of the stereochemistry of compound (7) at position 17 from β to α, and of compound (8) at position 20 from β to α markedly lowered potency (Ranade *et al.*, 1971; Kohen *et al.*, 1972). This work showed that potency was highest for compounds closest in structure to cholesterol.

All was not well, however, for studies in humans by Sachs and

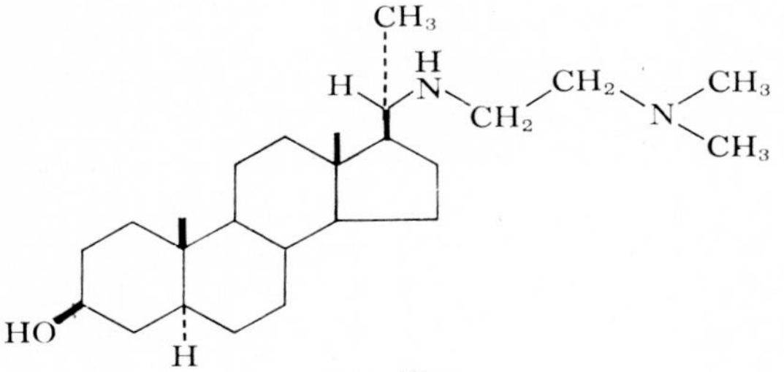
CH3
H
H
N
CH2
CH2
N
CH3
CH3
HO
H

(**1**)
22,25-Diazacholestanol

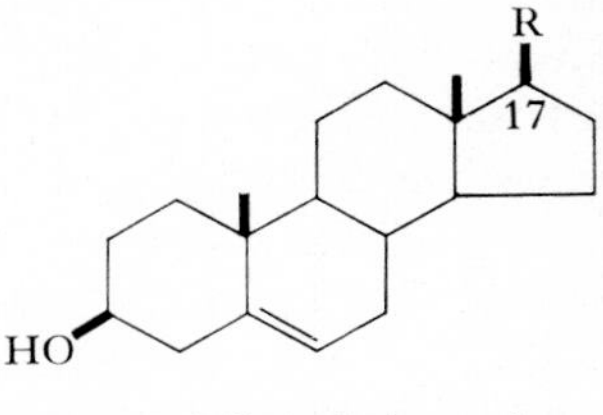
R
17
HO

Aza and diazacholesterols

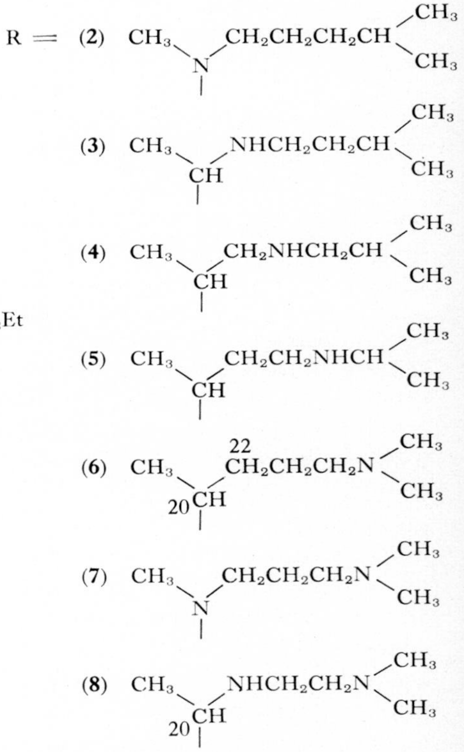
R =
(2) CH3 N CH2CH2CH2CH CH3 CH3
(3) CH3 CH NHCH2CH2CH CH3 CH3
(4) CH3 CH CH2NHCH2CH CH3 CH3
(5) CH3 CH CH2CH2NHCH CH3 CH3
(6) CH3 20 CH 22 CH2CH2CH2N CH3 CH3
(7) CH3 N CH2CH2CH2N CH3 CH3
(8) CH3 20 CH NHCH2CH2N CH3 CH3

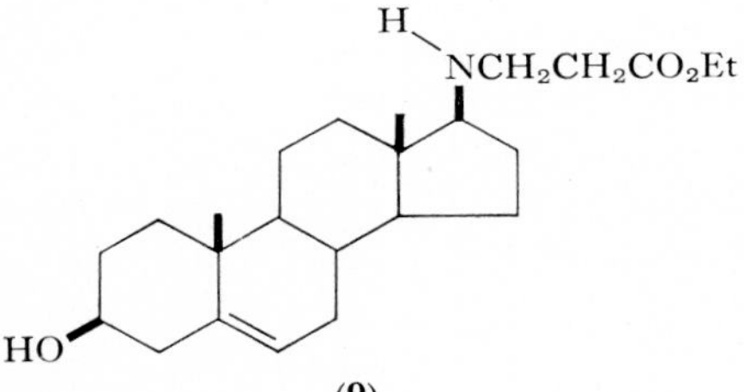
H
NCH2CH2CO2Et
HO

(**9**)

Wolfman (1962) and in rats by Dvornik and Kraml (1963) showed that the lowering of cholesterol was accompanied by a very significant increase in desmosterol, a cholesterol precursor which can be laid down in an atherosclerotic plaque. Because the fall in total sterol level was 9 per cent, there must have been some block before the squalene cyclization stage. Preliminary experiments suggested that 22,25-diazacholesterol (Ornitrol®) (**8**) reduced the rate of squalene cyclization to lanosterol (Ranney and Counsell, 1962). Gould and Swyrd (1966) have demonstrated that in the liver of rats fed cholesterol an enzyme between mevalonic acid and farnesyl pyrophosphate is inhibited, and probably the enzyme which converts farnesyl pyrophosphate to squalene.

The accumulation of desmosterol indicates blockade of cholesterol biosynthesis at the desmosterol-Δ^{24}-reductase stage. Later work by Niemiro and Fumagalli (1965) showed that 20,25-diazacholesterol (**7**) also inhibited 7-dehydrocholesterol-Δ^7-reductase in rat liver homogenate. It is possible that other analogues also inhibited that same enzyme, but at the time analytical techniques were not available for readily separating desmosterol and 7-dehydrocholesterol. In retrospect, it is perhaps not surprising that compounds close in structure to cholesterol will inhibit late stages in its biosynthesis.

The mechanism by which β-hydroxy-β-methylglutaryl-CoA reductase is altered by cholesterol feeding is still not understood completely. Cholesterol synthesis is not inhibited by addition of cholesterol to rat liver slices or homogenates, which suggests that cholesterol itself may not be the actual regulatory molecule. Siperstein and Fagan (1964) have suggested that a specific lipoprotein–cholesterol complex is the actual feedback inhibitor and that it acts directly, rather than by an inhibition of enzyme synthesis. On the other hand, Goldstein and Brown (1973) have shown that β-lipoproteins act as feedback inhibitors by suppressing synthesis of hydroxymethylglutaryl-CoA reductase. They have also suggested that familial hypercholesterolaemia (an example of type IIa) is caused by a complete absence of normal feedback suppression.

Figmonari and Rodwell (1965) have produced evidence that bile salts derived from cholesterol may be responsible for control of cholesterol biosynthesis. They inhibit the formation of mevalonate from acetate by rat liver homogenates. A bile acid analogue, the synthetic azacholenic acid derivative (**9**), has shown oral hypocholesterolaemic activity in rats (Venton *et al.*, 1973).

4.2 β-HYDROXY-β-METHYLGLUTARIC ACID

It has been suggested recently that β-hydroxy-β-methylglutaric acid (**10**), a natural metabolite formed in mammalian liver by the action of β-hydroxy-β-methylglutaryl-CoA hydrolase on β-hydroxy-β-methylglu-

$$\begin{array}{c} \text{Me} \\ | \\ \text{HO}_2\text{CCH}_2\text{CCH}_2\text{CO}_2\text{H} \\ | \\ \text{OH} \end{array}$$

(**10**)

taryl-CoA, may be a physiological metabolite responsible for regulating cholesterol synthesis. In rat liver slices and homogenates the compound inhibits the enzymic step mediated by β-hydroxy-β-methylglutaryl-CoA reductase, probably by a competitive mechanism (Beg and Lupien, 1972), and it lowers cholesterol levels in rats and in humans (Lupien *et al.*, 1973a). In rabbits it retards the establishment and progression of experimental atherosclerotic lesions. An increased rate of excretion of cholesterol may contribute to its action (Lupien *et al.*, 1973b).

4.3 NON-STEROIDAL INHIBITORS OF DESMOSTEROL-Δ^{24}-REDUCTASE AND 7-DEHYDROCHOLESTEROL-Δ^{7}-REDUCTASE.

Triparanol (MER 29®) **(11)**, an orally active hypocholesterolaemic agent (Blohm *et al.*, 1959), causes accumulation of desmosterol (Avigan *et al.*, 1960; Steinberg *et al.*, 1961), but because total sterol levels are reduced, there must also be a block at an earlier stage of the biosynthesis than desmosterol-Δ^{24}-reductase. It is thought to be at the cyclization of squalene stage. Triparanol also inhibits 7-dehydrocholesterol-Δ^{7}-reductase (Niemiro and Fumagalli, 1965). Triparanol was withdrawn from clinical work because at high doses it caused alopecia in several patients (Achor *et al.*, 1961). Both Triparanol and the related and more

(11)   Triparanol   (12)

Desmosterol-Δ^{24}-reductase inhibitors

potent acenaphthene **(12)** produced stillborn and abnormal foetuses in rats (Short *et al.*, 1965). There is no evidence to show that these side effects are related to the accumulation of desmosterol. Related compounds which block 7-dehydrocholesterol-Δ^{7}-reductase and cause 7-dehydrocholesterol to accumulate in plasma and tissues of treated rats are the benzimidazole **(13)** (Rodney *et al.*, 1965), the potent chloropyrimidine **(14)** (Bach *et al.*, 1967; Bach, 1970), and the even more potent compound boxidine **(15)** from the same group (Bach *et al.*, 1968). Although boxidine is shown as a Δ^{7}-reductase inhibitor, its main action is thought to be inhibition of reabsorption of 7-dehydrocholesterol from the bile (Gordon and Cekleniak, 1968), and so there is an absolute reduction in total

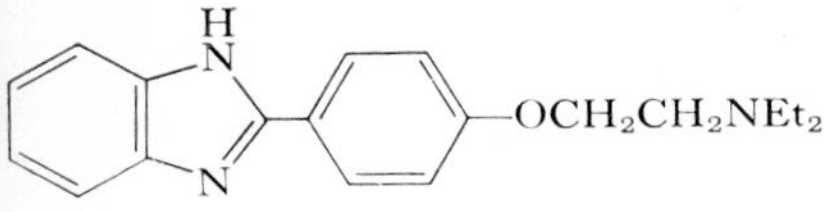

$-OCH_2CH_2NEt_2$

(13)

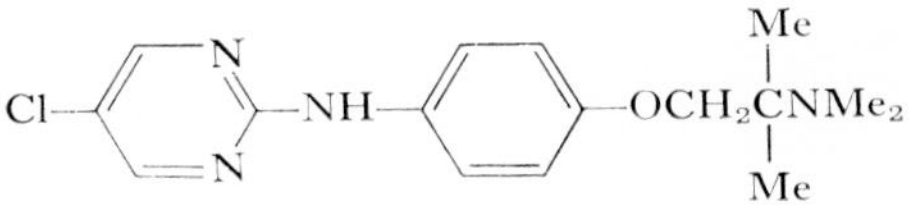

$Cl-\!\!\langle N \rangle\!\!-NH-\!\!\langle\ \rangle\!\!-OCH_2CNMe_2$ (Me, Me)

(14)

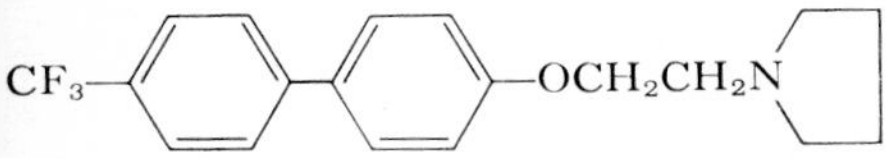

$CF_3-\!\!\langle\ \rangle\!\!-\!\!\langle\ \rangle\!\!-OCH_2CH_2N$

(15) Boxidine

$-CH_2NHCH_2-\!\!\langle\ \rangle\!\!---CH_2NHCH_2-$ (Cl ... Cl)

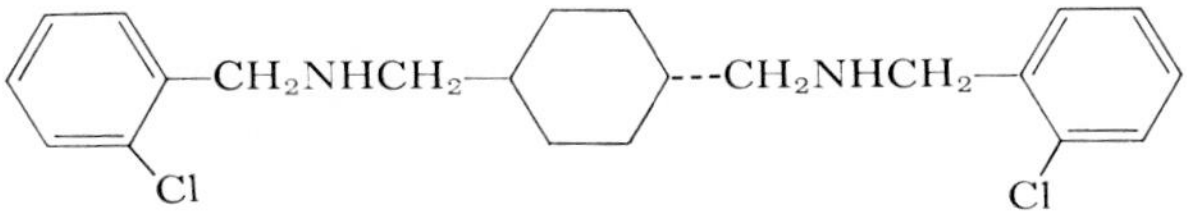

AY 9944

(16)

7–Dehydrocholesterol–Δ^7–reductase inhibitors

sterol. It reduces triglyceride and phospholipid levels in addition to cholesterol levels. AY 9944 (**16**) was developed from N,N'-dibenzylethyl-enediamine, which was being used to form salts of mevalonic acid ana-logues, and which was itself found to be an inhibitor of cholesterol bio-synthesis (Dvornik *et al.*, 1963: Humber *et al.*, 1966). AY 9944 does not inhibit the reduction of desmosterol (Niemiro and Fumagalli, 1965). It was found to have teratogenic properties in rats (Roux and Aubry, 1966).

4.4 FARNESOIC ACID ANALOGUES

The attraction of inhibiting the enzymic steps between mevalonate and squalene is mentioned above. Geranyl and farnesyl pyrophosphates are oxidized by liver enzymes to geranic (**17**) and farnesoic acids (**18**). These acids are not intermediates in cholesterol biosynthesis but are on cata-bolic pathways for removing intermediates. Popjak *et al.* (1960) have shown that farnesoic acid inhibits utilization of intermediates formed between mevalonate and squalene, and may be part of a physiological control mechanism. Several analogues were found to be effective inhibi-tors of cholesterol biosynthesis by rat liver homogenates, the best com-pound being the fully saturated derivative 3,7,11-trimethyldodecanoate (**19**). They inhibit mevalonic kinase, the enzyme which phosphorylates mevalonic acid. Piccinini (1962) has reported that farnesoic acid and some related compounds are not active in rats fed a normal or a fatty diet. However, Jouanneteau and Zwingelstein (1961) have reported that the

Geranyl pyrophosphate $\longrightarrow$

$$\underset{CH_3}{\overset{CH_3}{\diagdown}}C\!=\!CHCH_2CH_2\overset{\overset{\displaystyle CH_3}{|}}{C}\!=\!CHCO_2H$$

(**17**)   Geranic acid

Faresyl pyrophosphate $\longrightarrow$

$$\underset{CH_3}{\overset{CH_3}{\diagdown}}C\!=\!CHCH_2CH_2\overset{\overset{\displaystyle CH_3}{|}}{C}\!=\!CHCH_2CH_2\overset{\overset{\displaystyle CH_3}{|}}{C}\!=\!CHCO_2H$$

(**18**)   Farnesoic acid

$$\underset{CH_3}{\overset{CH_3}{\diagdown}}CHCH_2CH_2CH_2\overset{\overset{\displaystyle CH_3}{|}}{C}HCH_2CH_2CH_2\overset{\overset{\displaystyle CH_3}{|}}{C}HCH_2CO_2H$$

(**19**) 3,7,11-Trimethyldodecanoic acid

$$\underset{CH_3}{\overset{CH_3}{\diagdown}}C\!=\!CHCH_2CH_2\overset{\overset{\displaystyle CH_3}{|}}{C}\!=\!CHCH_2CH_2\overset{\overset{\displaystyle Et}{|}}{C}\!=\!CHCO_2H$$

(**20**)

farnesoic acid analogue (**20**) reduces serum and liver cholesterol in the rat. Its mode of action is not known. These compounds do not appear to have been developed further.

4.5   MEVALONIC ACID ANALOGUES

Certain analogues of mevalonic acid block enzymic steps between mevalonic acid and squalene. 3,5-Dihydroxy-3,4,4-trimethylvaleric acid (**21**) inhibits cholesterol biosynthesis by rat liver homogenates (Hulcher, 1971), but no *in vivo* studies have been reported. The accumulation of 5-phosphomevalonic acid suggests that the compound inhibits 5-phosphomevalonic kinase.

The next enzyme in the biosynthetic sequence, mevalonic pyrophosphate decarboxylase, is inhibited by 2-fluoromevalonic acid (**22**). That compound has two asymmetric centres, but of the four optical isomers only one could act as a substrate for first mevalonic kinase and then 5-phosphomevalonic kinase. The resulting 2-fluoromevalonic acid 5-pyrophosphate (**23**) was not a substrate for the decarboxylase enzyme, and moreover it inhibited the decarboxylation of mevalonic acid 5-pyrophosphate to isopentenyl pyrophosphate (Kirschner *et al.*, 1961). The analogue (**24**) containing a fluoromethyl group was found to inhibit the incorporation of acetate by rat liver enzymes some 5 to 10 times more effectively than incorporation of mevalonate, and so this compound must inhibit a pre-mevalonate step (Singer *et al.*, 1959). These compounds have not been developed, possibly because they lack potency in mammalian systems. Perhaps the compounds never reach the site of action because of metabolism or distribution characteristics.

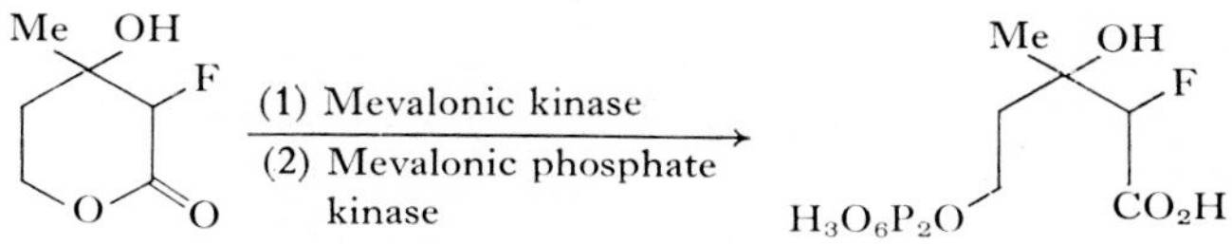

(22) 2-Fluoromevalonic acid lactone

(23)

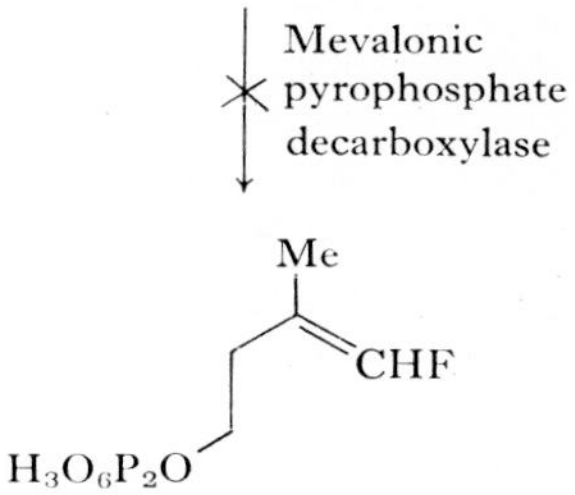

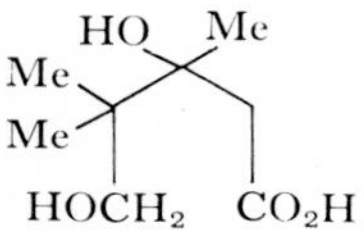

(21)

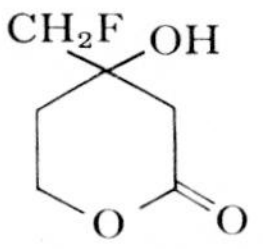

(24) 3-Fluoromethyl-3-hydroxyvalerolactone

4.6 BENZMALECENE

An unrelated compound considered to block between mevalonate and squalene is benzmalecene (25) (Baer *et al.*, 1959; Huff and Gilfillan, 1960). Addition of benzmalecene to rat liver homogenates caused the

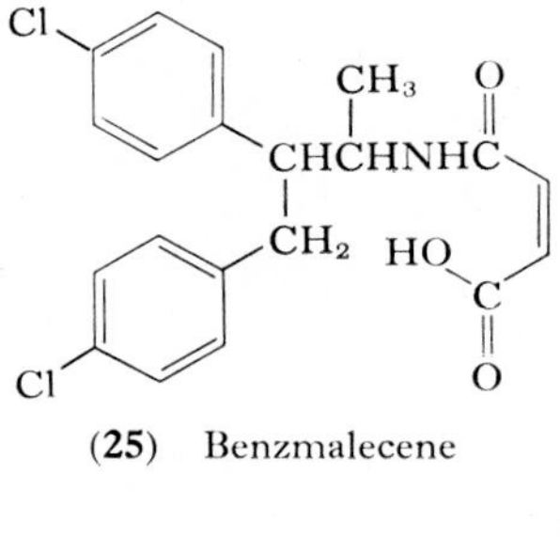

(25) Benzmalecene

accumulation of large amounts of polyisoprenoids (Holmes and DiTullio, 1962). It effectively reduced cholesterol levels in humans, but in some there was a significant rise in triglyceride levels, suggesting that there was also a pre-mevalonate block. This would lead to an increase in intermediates for fatty acid biosynthesis (Page and Schneckloth, 1959).

Benzmalecene also inhibited active absorption of bile acids by the small intestine (Lack and Weiner, 1963). It was withdrawn because of liver toxicity (Page and Schneckloth, 1959).

4.7 OESTROGENS

Oestrogens lower serum cholesterol and β-lipoprotein levels in man, and increase the lipid content of pre-β-lipoproteins (Furman *et al.*, 1967; 1968). This increase may be related to an observed decrease in post-heparin lipolytic activity and impaired plasma triglyceride removal (Hazzard *et al.*, 1969). Oestrogens may in fact aggravate hyperlipidaemic conditions.

Hypocholesterolaemic properties can be retained and oestrogenic effects minimized by chemical manipulation of the basic oestrogen structure. The dihydrocinnamate ester (26) has little oestrogenic activity in rats (Arnold *et al.*, 1966), but no effects on lipids in man have been disclosed. The mechanism by which oestrogens affect lipid metabolism is not known, although some effects on cholesterol biosynthesis have been recorded. 16,16-Difluoroequilenin methyl ether (27) inhibits the incorporation of mevalonic acid into cholesterol by rat liver enzymes (Humber *et al.*, 1962). In liver homogenates from rats given oral oestrone at a hypocholesterolaemic dose incorporation of mevalonic acid into sterols was less than in controls, and the block was shown to be at a stage or stages between mevalonic acid and isopentenyl pyrophosphate (Merola and Arnold, 1964). However, Mukherjee and Bhose (1968) suggest that 17β-oestradiol inhibits a pre-mevalonate step or steps. The diethylaminoethyl ether of oestradiol (28) inhibits the reduction of desmosterol to cholesterol in rat liver (Hughes *et al.*, 1964).

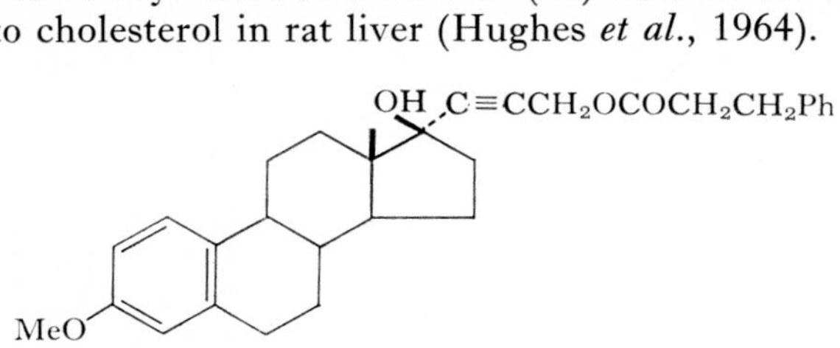

OH C≡CCH₂OCOCH₂CH₂Ph

MeO

(26)

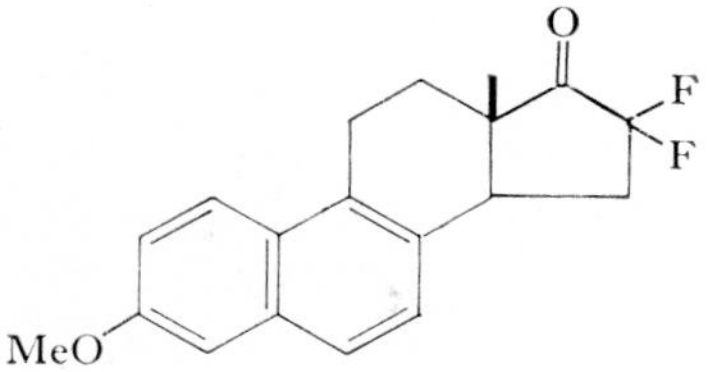

(27)

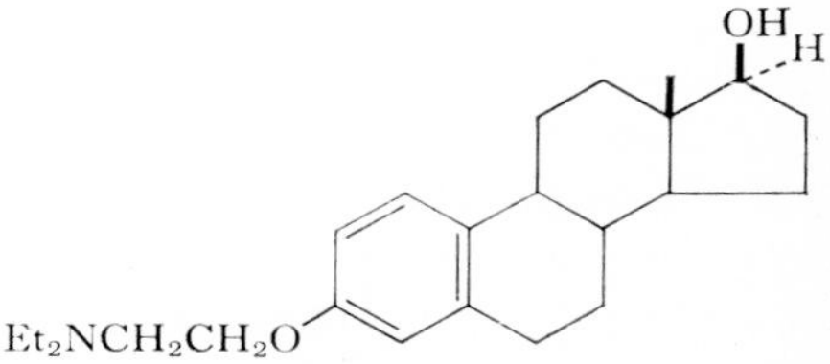

(28)

The oestrogen Premarin was withdrawn from The Coronary Drug Project (1970) at the 5 mg per day level because of a significantly increased incidence of cardiac events compared with the placebo group.

4.8 ARYLALKANOIC ACIDS

α-Phenylbutyric acid (29) lowers serum cholesterol levels in rats (Cottet *et al.*, 1953), but not in humans according to Fredrickson and Steinberg (1957). It inhibits *in vitro* synthesis of both cholesterol and fatty acids from acetate, acting at the stage at which free acetate is activated to acetyl-CoA. Because glucose and fatty acids can give rise to acetyl-CoA without the intervention of free acetate, the compound need have no effect on cholesterol synthesis from these major precursors. The related α-biphenylylbutyric acid (30) and difenesic acid (31) inhibit at some stage after mevalonic acid formation (Tavormina and Gibbs, 1957; Morand *et al.*, 1964).

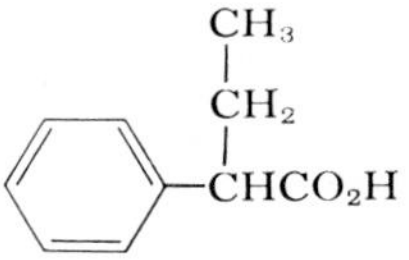

(29)

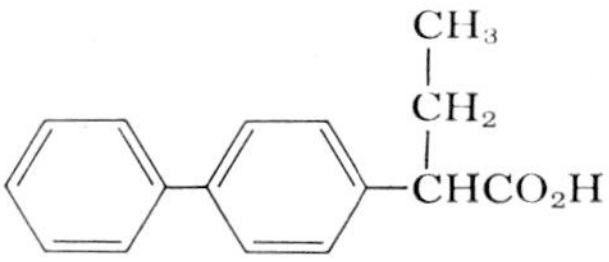

(30)

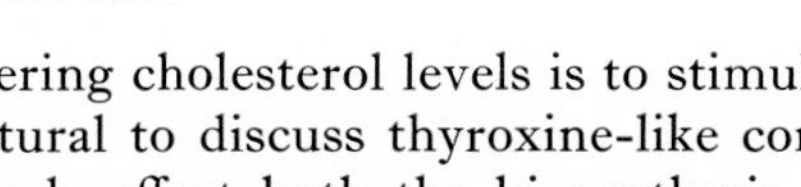

(31) Difenesic acid

4.9 THYROXINE ANALOGUES

Another way of lowering cholesterol levels is to stimulate the removal of cholesterol. It is natural to discuss thyroxine-like compounds first, because such compounds affect both the biosynthesis and catabolism of cholesterol, and because they provide a link with the clofibrate-type compounds in the next section. Thyroxine (32) increases the rate of cholesterol biosynthesis in the liver but at the same time it increases proportionally more the rate of removal of cholesterol and its metabolites (Kritchevsky, 1964). Thyroxine increases the rate of cholesterol biosynthesis from acetate but not from mevalonate and so its effect on biosynthesis is pre-mevalonate (Fletcher and Myant, 1958; 1960). Low

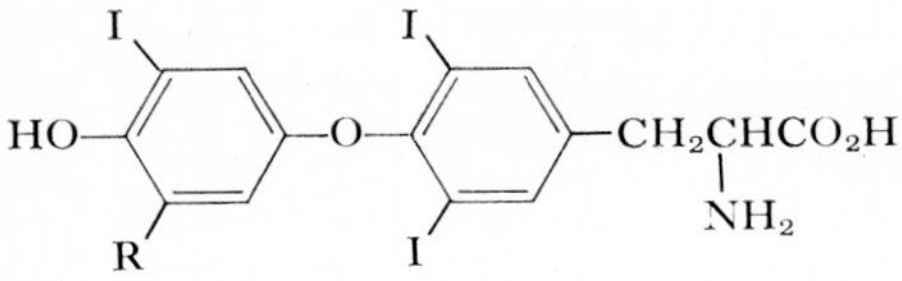

(32) R = I = Thyroxine
(33) R = H = Triiodothyronine

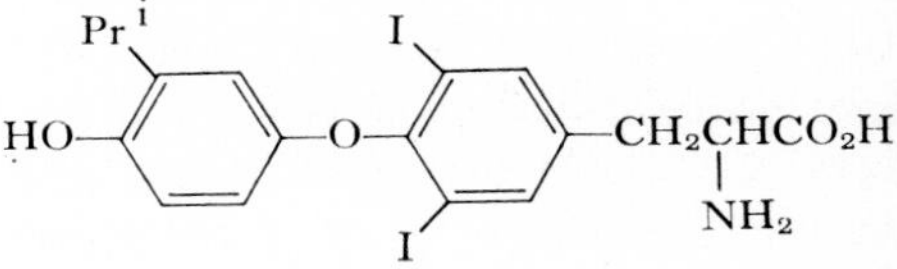

(34)

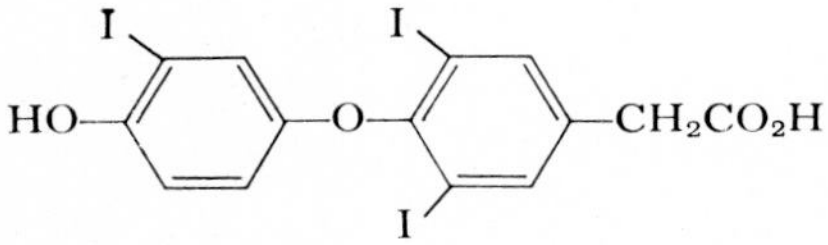

(35)

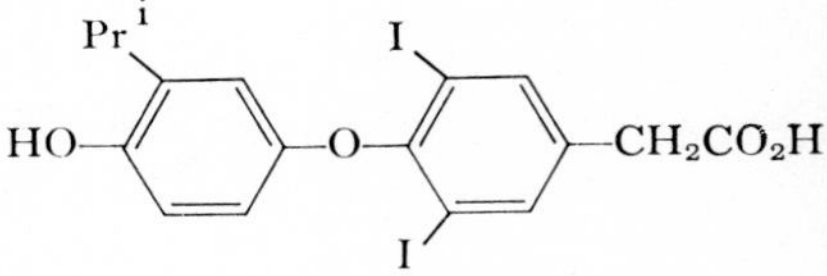

(36)

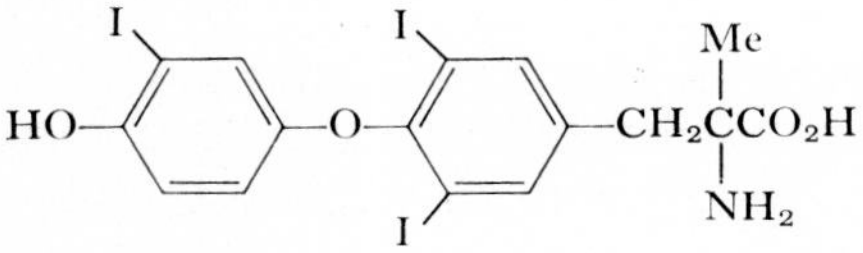

(37)

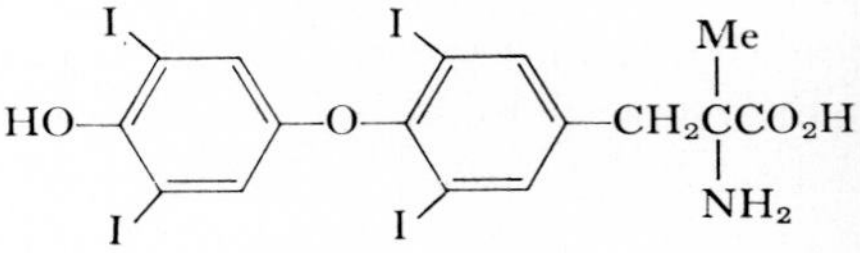

(38)

levels of thyroxine raise the levels of β-hydroxy-β-methylglutaryl-CoA reductase by causing synthesis of new enzyme, for which there is an induction period (Guder *et al.*, 1968). It is interesting to note that higher levels of thyroxine inhibit that same enzyme, controlling its activity so that too much acetyl-CoA is not shunted from the general body pool (Eskelson *et al.*, 1970). The enzymic step or steps in the degradation and excretion of cholesterol which are stimulated by thyroxine are not known. Mitropoulos and Myant (1965) suggest that it stimulates a rate-limiting reaction leading to cleavage of the side chain of cholesterol, but that it has little or no influence on the hydroxylations of the ring system.

The aim of the medicinal chemist has been to try to dissociate the hypolipidaemic action of thyroxine analogues from their calorigenic and cardiotropic effects. L-Tri-iodothyronine (**33**) is more potent then L-thyroxine and has tended to be used as a standard for comparison. Blank *et al.* (1963; 1964) reported that the analogue (**34**) was slightly more potent, and analogues (**35**) and (**36**) somewhat less potent than L-tri-iodothyronine as lipid-lowering agents, and that they showed better separation of desirable and undesirable properties. The separation was not enough, however, because compound (**35**) displayed undesirable side effects in clinical trials. The replacement of iodine by isopropyl is interesting from a physicochemical point of view (Hansch and Fujita, 1964). The methyl ethers of compounds (**35**) and (**36**) show an even greater separation of properties but they do not seem to have been followed up in the clinic. Both L- and D-thyroxine have hypolipidaemic activity, and in the case of the D-isomer useful activity seemed sufficiently dissociated from undesirable metabolic properties to permit its clinical use. Until 1972 it was one of the four drugs being examined by The Coronary Drug Project Research Group (1972). However, it can affect the heart adversely and it has been withdrawn from the Project because of excess mortality associated with the drug. Hughes and Moore (1967) examined some α-methyl analogues of thyroxine in rats and concluded that D-α-methyltri-iodothyronine (**37**) would have less tendency to induce symptoms of calorigenic activity than D-thyroxine at equally hypolipaemic doses. Blank *et al.* (1966) had independently looked at DL-α-methylthyroxine (**38**) and showed that it had weak cholesterol lowering activity. However, Beckmann and co-workers (1972) have shown that the ethyl ester of (**38**) (CG 635) has a good separation of lipid lowering and basal metabolic effects in rats, and have pressed on with clinical work (Ditschuneit *et al.*, 1972; Gries *et al.*, 1972). It lowers cholesterol levels by about 20 per cent at 40 mg per day orally in types II, IV, and V lipidaemias without significant changes in body weight or calorigenic action.

4.10   ARYLOXYALKANOIC ACIDS

4.10.1   *Clofibrate and certain close analogues*

There is intense clinical and biochemical interest in clofibrate (Atromid-S®) (39), which lowers pre-β-lipoprotein (triglyceride) and β-lipoprotein (cholesterol) levels in man, and which is being examined in The Coronary Drug Project (US Public Health Service, 1967). One aspect of the mode of action of clofibrate, which is hydrolysed to the acid *in vivo*, is dependent in part on thyroxine (Platt and Thorp, 1966). Clofibrate displaces thyroxine from its binding sites on albumin and the displaced thyroxine is selectively taken up by the liver. Thus, the liver becomes relatively hyperthyroid and for the reasons already given for thyroxine, a contribution could be made to the lowering of serum cholesterol levels. Mitochondrial preparations from livers of clofibrate-fed rats show an increased capacity to oxidize cholesterol to carbon dioxide (Kritchevsky *et al.*, 1969), but 7α-hydroxylation of cholesterol by liver microsomes is unaffected (Einarsson *et al.*, 1974). Since, at a dose level which lowers lipids, clofibrate fails to enter rat liver cells, it is unlikely that effects on the liver are direct effects (Platt and Thorp, 1966).

(39)   Clofibrate

(40)   Methyl clofenapate   (41)   ICI 55,897

However, the extra-hepatic effects of clofibrate are quite different from those of thyroxine, which stimulates the release of free fatty acid from adipose tissue (Fisher and Ball, 1967). Either tissues other than the liver become relatively hypothyroid or some effect which overrides thyroxine must operate. Barrett (1966) has shown that clofibrate produces a marked reduction in the rate of fatty acid release from rat adipose tissue incubated in plasma. In accordance with that, decreased adenyl cyclase activity has been found for adipose tissue from clofibrate-treated rats (Greene *et al.*, 1970), a result confirmed *in vitro* by Carlson *et al.* (1972). Numerous investigators have suggested that the inhibition of fatty acid mobilization *in vivo* is responsible for at least a part of the hypotriglyceridaemic effect of clofibrate (Witiak *et al.*, 1971a). In line with the above observation, the effect of clofibrate on cholesterol levels is reduced by thyroidectomy (Best and Duncan, 1964) and the effects on cholesterol and triglycerides are abolished by hypophysectomy (Thorp, 1963). Irrespective of mechanism, clofibrate has a limited thyroxine-like effect which alters lipid metabolism without being calorigenic (Westerfeld *et al.*, 1968). The result of the redistribution of plasma-protein bound compounds such as thyroxine into the liver is a disturbance of the metabolic equilibrium of the cell, which changes until a new balance is attained. The new balance is then maintained throughout drug treatment. Rat liver weight is increased (hepatomegaly) by clofibrate, and liver protein concentrations are raised (Platt and Thorp, 1966). Hepatocytes are larger than normal. The levels of pyridine nucleotide coenzymes and the activity of several dependent dehydrogenases are raised in the period of the new equilibrium (Platt and Cockrill, 1966). Microbody (peroxisome) proliferation is increased, and this is associated with an elevation of catalase activity resulting from an increased rate of synthesis of the enzyme (Reddy *et al.*, 1973). The relatively wasteful enzymic activity of peroxisomes (de Duve and Baudhuin, 1966) could result in less efficient conversion of dietary and depot substrates to carbohydrate and lipid in the liver, heat being produced rather than glycogen or lipoprotein. Liver size returns to normal after withdrawal of clofibrate. It is not known whether hepatomegaly is produced in humans given the conventional clinical dosage of clofibrate, which on a weight basis is only one tenth of the dose which causes hepatomegaly in rats.

In addition to the displacement of thyroxine mentioned above, the acid corresponding to clofibrate also displaces fatty acids from their binding sites on albumin (Thorp, 1971). Desaminothyroxine was used as a biochemical probe for fatty acid binding sites. Fatty acids displaced from strong to weaker binding sites on albumin would be more readily available for uptake and utilization by cells and so lower amounts would reach the liver (Spector and Soboroff, 1971). The uptake of fatty acids into cells would be helped by an increase in carnitine acyltransferase activity as noted by Solberg *et al.* (1972) for rats fed clofibrate. The drug does lower the absolute circulating concentrations of free fatty acids in both rats and dogs (Barrett and Thorp, 1968). As a result of the perturbed transport of free fatty acid and also of the inhibition of lipolysis in adipose tissue noted above, the availability of fatty acid to the liver for triglyceride and pre-β-lipoprotein synthesis would be reduced.

Thorp and his colleagues have found compounds which show selectivity in displacing thyroxine or desaminothyroxine from their binding sites on albumin. The acid corresponding to clofibrate displaces both thyroxine and desaminothyroxine from their binding sites on human albumin and in the clinic lowers cholesterol levels and even more so lowers triglyceride levels. It is particularly effective in patients with type III and type IV hyperlipidaemias (Blohm, 1973). The acid corresponding to methyl clofenapate (**40**) (Thorp, 1970) displaces thyroxine from its binding sites rather than desaminothyroxine, and if the displacement mechanism was solely responsible for its activity the compound would be expected to have a greater effect on cholesterol levels relative to triglyceride levels than does clofibrate. In those patients treated with the compound that did appear to be so (Craig and Walton, 1972; Craig, 1972). Its effect on triglycerides could arise in part by a mechanism other than that involving displacement of fatty acids from binding sites. It is a more potent inhibitor of acetyl-CoA carboxylase than clofibrate (Maragoudakis, 1970). Methyl clofenapate was withdrawn because of delayed liver toxicity in rodents (Craig, 1972), although adverse effects on the liver had not been seen in patients. Clinical examination of the compound ICI 55,897 (**41**) is just beginning (Thorp, 1973). This compound selectively displaces desaminothyroxine rather than thyroxine from binding sites on human albumin and based on the displacement theory is expected to have a greater effect than clofibrate on triglyceride levels relative to cholesterol levels. According to the displacement theory, this compound should have little effect directly attributable to thyroxine displacement on serum cholesterol levels. It may provide support for thyroxine displacement being involved in cholesterol lowering by clofibrate.

Clofibrate has many actions in addition to those mentioned above, and it is not possible at this stage to say with certainty which of its effects are crucial for its biological action. Its actions have been summarized recently by Blohm (1973) and by Havel and Kane (1973). They include inhibition of acetyl-CoA carboxylase, the enzyme which catalyses the formation of malonyl-CoA, the first committed step and possibly rate-limiting step in fatty acid biosynthesis (Maragoudakis et al., 1972). Interruption of lipid synthesis at this stage should not lead to the accumulation of undesirable intermediates because acetyl-CoA can be directed into the citric acid cycle. In mitochondria from livers of clofibrate-fed rats, acetoacetyl-CoA deacylase activity is stimulated, thus aiding removal of an intermediate in lipid biosynthesis (Burch and Curran, 1969).

β-Hydroxy-β-methylglutaryl-CoA reductase activity is reduced in the liver of rats fed clofibrate (White, 1971), and acetate activation is impaired, although as discussed earlier the latter action need have no effect on lipid biosynthesis. The effect on the reductase activity is opposite to that expected, based on the thyroxine displacement theory, but attention is drawn to the comments of Eskelson et al. (1970) on the effects of different levels of thyroxine on β-hydroxy-β-methylglutaryl-CoA reductase. Conversion of mevalonic acid to mevalonic acid 5-phosphate by bovine aorta cell free systems is inhibited by clofibrate (Walsh *et al.*, 1969). Azarnoff *et al.* (1965) have shown that in the liver of clofibrate fed rats a step between mevalonic acid and isopentenyl pyrophosphate is inhibited. Earlier work *in vitro* had indicated a site of inhibition between squalene and lanosterol.

Inhibition of rat liver microsomal preparations of glycerol-3-phosphate acyltransferase, the enzyme which begins triglyceride synthesis, has been reported (Fallon *et al.*, 1971; Lamb and Fallon, 1972), and also stimulation of glycerol-3-phosphate dehydrogenase activity (Westerfeld *et al.*, 1968). The latter effect, which is characteristic of thyroxine, would decrease the amount of glycerol-3-phosphate available for triglyceride synthesis by converting it into dihydroxyacetone phosphate. The availability of glycerol-3-phosphate may also be reduced by inhibition of the glycolytic enzymes glucose-6-phosphate dehydrogenase and fructose-1,6-diphosphate aldolase by clofibrate (Zakin *et al.*, 1970; Maragoudakis *et al.*, 1972). Inhibition of glycolytic enzymes may be doubly useful because Weber *et al.* (1966) have shown that the hepatic level of free fatty acid operates a feedback control on the extent to which glycolytic pathways are used. Glycolysis would be enhanced by low availability of free fatty acids. Inhibition of palmitoyl-CoA deacylase in rat liver microsomes by clofibrate may raise cellular concentrations of palmitoyl-CoA to levels which could inhibit acetyl-CoA carboxylase and glycerol-3-phosphate acyl transferase (Lamb *et al.*, 1973).

Dietary clofibrate increases the action of rat adipose tissue lipoprotein lipase, the enzyme responsible for removing triglycerides from chylomicrons and pre-β-lipoproteins (Tolman *et al.*, 1970). That process could be helped by the increase in activity of triglyceride synthesizing enzymes in clofibrate-fed rat adipose tissue noted by Giocoli *et al.* (1971), an increase which may be related to the enhanced uptake of fatty acids by adipose tissue shown to occur *in vitro* by Nestel and Austin (1968). The increased action of lipoprotein lipase may result indirectly. In man, Strisower *et al.* (1965) found that clofibrate increases the amount of α-lipoprotein polypeptide components (same concentration of α-lipoprotein with reduced triglyceride content), and α-lipoprotein polypeptide, which is transferred to convert nascent pre-β-lipoprotein to pre-β-lipoprotein (p. 8), functions as a cofactor for lipoprotein lipase (LaRosa *et al.*, 1970; Havel *et al.*, 1970). However, clofibrate inhibits human serum lipoprotein lipase *in vitro* at concentrations which start four times greater than the therapeutic concentration *in vivo* (Whayne and Witiak, 1973). The effect may be non-specific.

Grundy *et al.* (1972) have reported that clofibrate mobilizes cholesterol from tissue stores.

4.10.2   *Other aryloxyalkanoic acids*

Other aryloxyacid derivates related to clofibrate are of interest. Like clofibrate, nafenopin (Melipan®) (**42**) has a greater effect on serum triglycerides than on serum cholesterol (Hess and Bencze, 1968; Dujovne *et al.*, 1971). Nikkila and Kekki (1972) have shown that it reduces the production of plasma triglycerides in man. Like clofibrate, it inhibits acetyl-CoA carboxylase *in vitro* (Maragoudakis, 1969). There was a decrease in activity of the glycolytic enzymes fructose 6-phosphate kinase and pyruvate kinase, and citrate cleavage enzyme was suppressed in rats dosed with nafenopin (Schacht and Granzer, 1970). It produces hepatomegaly in rats at a lower dosage level than clofibrate (Best and Duncan, 1970), and catalase activity is increased (Reddy *et al.*, 1973). Liver mitochondrial preparations from rats fed nafenopin show increased ability to oxidize cholesterol relative to preparations from control animals (Kritchevsky and Tepper, 1969). Nafenopin was withdrawn because of liver damage in rats on long-term high dose studies (Russo and Mendlowitz, 1971). Some signs of liver toxity were seen in the clinic (Katterman *et al.*, 1972).

Halofenate (**43**) markedly lowers serum triglyceride and uric acid levels, but has little effect on cholesterol levels (Sirtori *et al.*, 1971; Jepson *et al.*, 1972). The free acid from halofenate displaces thyroxine from plasma thyroxine-binding globulin (Morgan *et al.*, 1971), and halofenate enhances cholesterol oxidation by rat liver mitochondria (Kritchevsky and Tepper, 1972). It produces hepatomegaly in the rat (Gilfillan *et al.*, 1971). Like clofibrate it displaces fatty acids from strong to weaker binding sites on albumin and increases fatty acid uptake into mammalian cells (Spector and Soboroff, 1971).

SaH 42-348 (**44**) which reduces all serum lipids in rats (Timms *et al.*, 1969) does not have a significant effect on cholesterol biosynthesis and it was thought to act by increasing cholesterol catabolism (Kelly and Ho, 1969). Kritchevsky and Tepper (1973) have shown that it does not enhance cholesterol oxidation and have suggested that the marked reduction in weight gain of the treated rats may explain some of the lipid lowering effects. It causes hepatomegaly in rats (Timms *et al.*, 1968).

AT-308 (**45**) is a potent hypocholesterolaemic agent which shows little effect on triglyceride levels. It inhibits hepatic cholesterol biosynthesis from acetate but not from mevalonate, and does not inhibit mobilization of fatty acid from adipose tissue (Imai *et al.*, 1973).

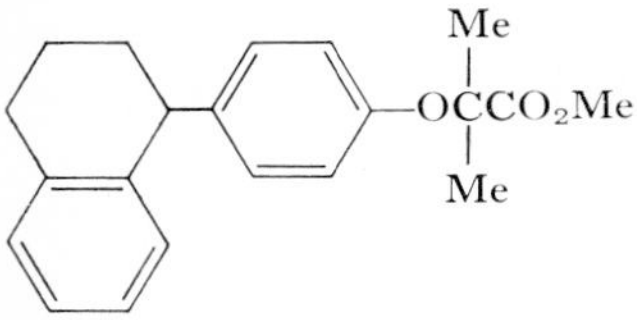

(**42**) Nafenopin (Su-13437)

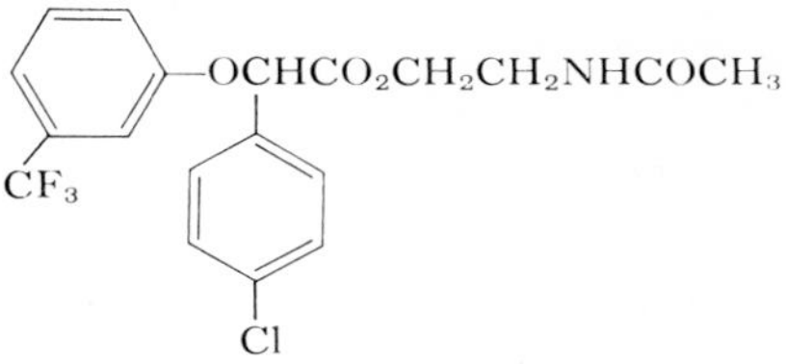

(**43**) Halofenate (MK 185)

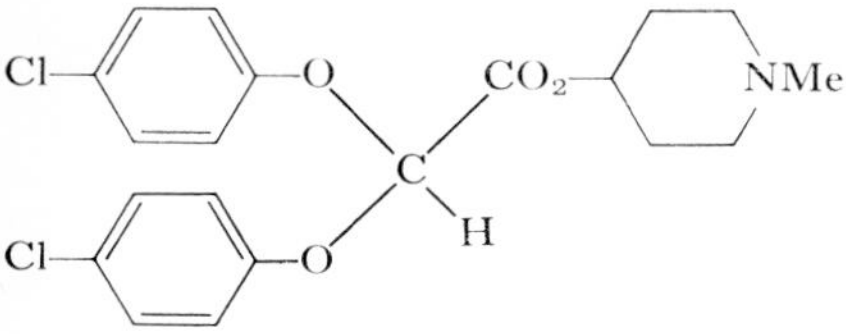

(**44**) SaH 42-348

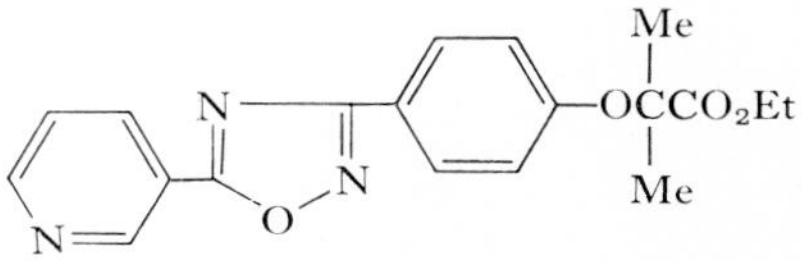

(**45**) AT-308

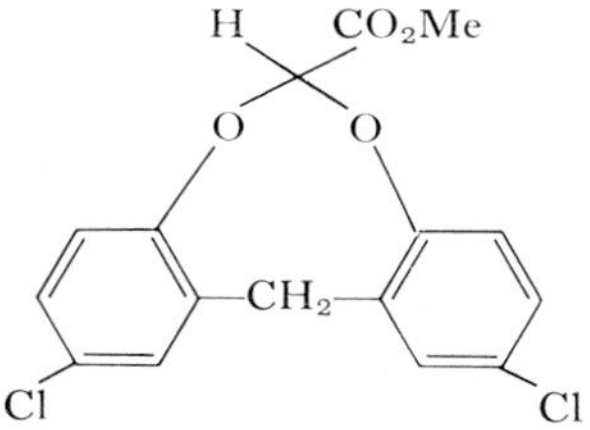

(**46**) Treloxinate

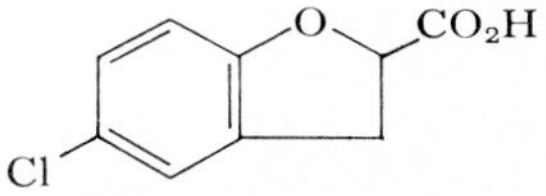

(**47**)

Treloxinate (**46**) is more potent than clofibrate in lowering cholesterol and triglycerides (Kariya *et al.*, 1972; Grisar *et al.*, 1972). In the rat it inhibits hepatic synthesis of cholesterol from acetate, but not from mevalonate, and it enhances oxidation of cholesterol. Other cyclic aryloxy acids related to clofibrate, e.g. (**47**), have been investigated, particularly for their effects on mobilization of free fatty acid from rat adipose tissue *in vitro* (Witiak *et al.*, 1971a). These authors conclude that the hypolipidaemic and hypocholesterolaemic effects of clofibrate are dissociated.

4.11 NICOTINIC ACID

Nicotinic acid (**48**) is used widely in the clinic in high doses to lower cholesterol and triglyceride levels, and is one of the drugs in The Coronary Drug Project (US Public Health Service, 1967). It lowers β-lipoprotein

levels and is particularly useful in patients with severe type IIa hyperlipidaemia (Levy and Rifkind, 1973). Its main action is to inhibit the
mobilization of free fatty acid from adipose tissue (Carlson and Orö,
1962), thus reducing fatty acid turnover and availability of fatty acid for
triglyceride synthesis in the liver. As a result less β-lipoprotein will need
to be synthesized to transport triglycerides from the liver, and ultimately
plasma β-lipoprotein levels will be lower than they would have been if
fatty acid mobilization had not been inhibited. Thus, lowering of serum
cholesterol levels is secondary to inhibition of fatty acid mobilization.
Inhibition of mobilization is mediated by inhibition of the enzyme
adenyl cyclase (Skidmore et al., 1971). There are conflicting reports

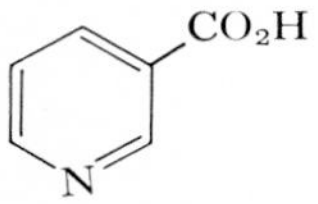

(48)

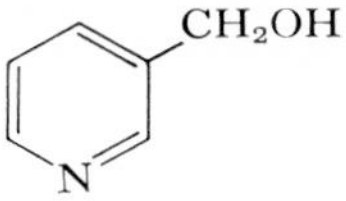

(49)

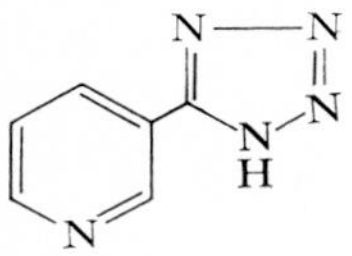

(50)

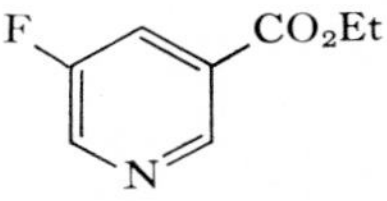

(51)

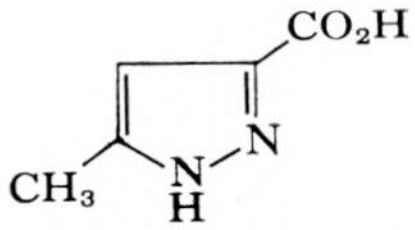

(52)   U-19425

concerning the effect of nicotinic acid on cholesterol biosynthesis
(Kritchevsky, 1971). Although in vitro it enhances oxidative removal of
the cholesterol side chain, a step involved in bile acid production
(Kritchevsky and Tepper, 1962), it does not appear to increase bile acid
excretion in patients (Kritchevsky, 1971). Nicotinic acid has also been
shown to mobilize cholesterol from body pools and to increase excretion
of neutral sterols (Miettinen, 1968).

Related hypolipidaemic compounds which inhibit lipolysis are the
corresponding alcohol (49) (Zöllner and Gudenzi, 1967), which is metabolized to nicotinic acid, the analogue in which the carboxylic acid
group has been replaced by the acidic tetrazole ring system (50) (Pereira
et al., 1968), 5-fluoronicotinic ester (51) (Carlson et al., 1969), and

5-methylpyrazole-3-carboxylic acid (52) (Kupiecki and Marshall, 1968). Other analogues inhibit fatty acid synthesis from acetate and cholesterol synthesis from mevalonate in rat liver (Hamilton *et al.*, 1971).

4.12 ANABOLIC-ANDROGENIC AGENTS

Many testosterone analogues lower both chylomicron and pre-β-lipoprotein triglycerides in hypertriglyceridaemic patients. The precise mechanism of action is not known. Oxandrolone (53) markedly stimulates post-heparin lipolytic activity which is reflected in increases in triglyceride lipase and monoglyceride hydrolase activity. Increased peripheral triglyceride hydrolysis may in part account for its triglyceride lowering effect (Glueck, 1971). Other studies suggest that these agents may have a thyromimetic action. For example, PS179 (54) increases the rate of oxidation of cholesterol to bile acids in male bile-fistula rats. However, it decreases the rate of incorporation of acetate into liver cholesterol (Nakamura *et al.*, 1967).

(53)   Oxandrolone   (54)   PS179

4.13 INHIBITORS OF CHOLESTEROL ABSORPTION

Four compounds which are considered to act mainly by inhibiting absorption or reabsorption of cholesterol from the intestine are the linoleamide, AC 223 (Clinolamide®) (55) (Fukushima *et al.*, 1969), β-sitosterol (56) (Gould, 1955), 5α-cholestane-3β,5α,6β-triol (57) (Imai *et al.*, 1967), and probucol (Biphenabid®) (58) (Miettinen, 1972; Nash, 1972; Polachek *et al.*, 1972).

The linoleamide does not affect cholesterol synthesis or side-chain oxidation *in vitro* (Kritchevsky and Tepper, 1971). Its effect on absorption may be related to its ability to form a complex with cholesterol. The linoleic acid portion of the molecule can be transferred to cholesterol *in vitro* to give an unsaturated ester of less sclerogenic potential, but this transfer was not observed *in vivo* (Abdulla and Adams, 1971).

It has been noted that when the cholestanetriol is fed to rabbits, lesions are produced in the aorta which resemble human lesions much

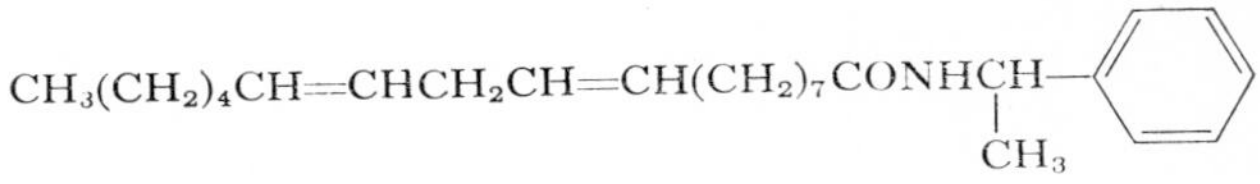
CH3(CH2)4CH=CHCH2CH=CH(CH2)7CONHCH
CH3

(**55**) Linolexamide (AC 223)

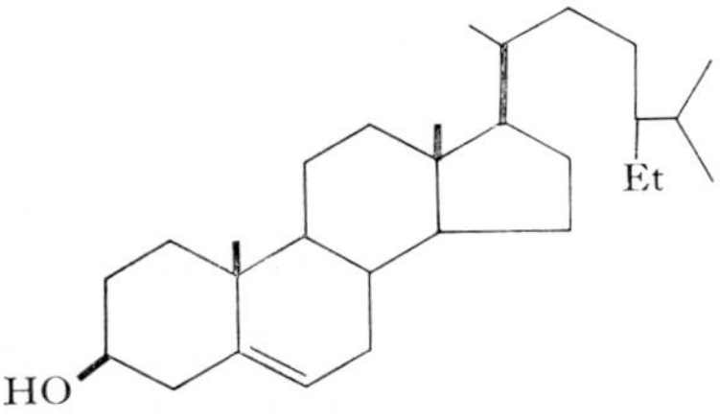
Et
HO

(**56**) β-Sitosterol

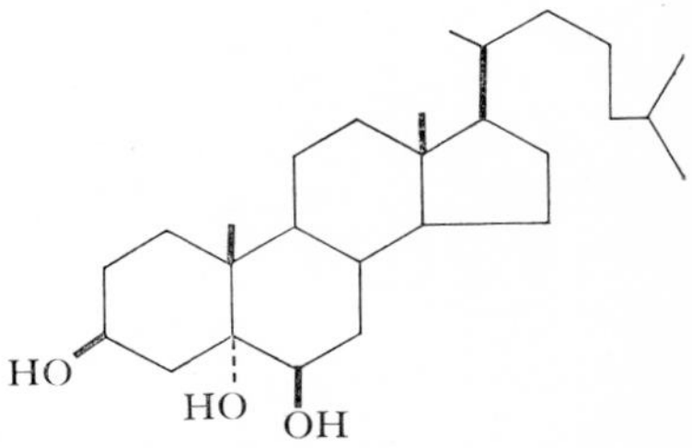
HO
HO
OH

(**57**) 5α-Cholestane-3β,5α,6β-triol

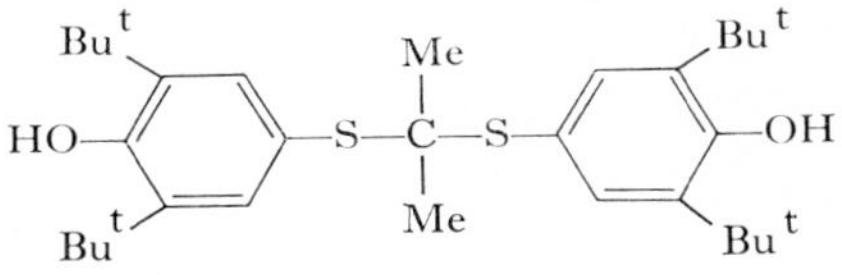
Bu^t
Me
Bu^t
HO
S
C
S
OH
Bu^t
Me
Bu^t

(**58**) Probucol (DH 581)

more than those produced by feeding cholesterol, and it has been suggested that it may be the etiological agent in man (Cook and MacDougall, 1968). The cholestanetriol inhibits the incorporation of acetate, mevalonate, and squalene into non-saponifiable products *in vitro* and causes accumulation of a new 29-30 C-atom sterol intermediate in the cholesterol biosynthesis pathway. The enzymes Δ^7-sterol Δ^5-dehydrogenase and $\Delta^{5,7}$-sterol Δ^7-reductase are inhibited (Witiak *et al.*, 1971b).

Other suggested modes of action for probucol are inhibition of cholesterol biosynthesis between acetate and mevalonate (Parsons, 1972), inhibition of free fatty acid release from rat adipose tissue, inhibition of release of lipoprotein cholesterol from the liver (Barnhart *et al.*, 1972), and increase in bile acid excretion (Miettinen, 1972).

Inhibition of 7-dehydrocholesterol reabsorption by boxidine (**15**) has been mentioned earlier.

4.14 BILE ACID BINDING AGENTS

Cholestyramine (MK 135) (Havel and Kane, 1973), Colestipol (U-26,597A) (Parkinson *et al.*, 1970) and Diethylaminoethyl-Sephadex

(Howard and Hyams, 1971) are bile acid binding resins which are not absorbed from the intestine themselves, but which prevent reabsorption of bile acids and thus increase their faecal excretion. Since bile acids inhibit the rate limiting 7α-hydroxylation of cholesterol (Mosbach, 1969), sequestraion of bile acid increases the oxidative removal of cholesterol. But removal of cholesterol removes a negative feedback inhibition to β-hydroxy-β-methylglutaryl-CoA reductase, and so cholesterol biosynthesis is increased (White, 1972). Hepatic cholesterol synthesis can increase sufficiently to compensate for its loss through increased oxidation to bile acids (Goodman and Noble, 1968; Moutafis and Myant, 1969). Levy et al. (1972) carried out labelling studies on β-lipoprotein and suggested that cholestyramine acts by increasing the catabolic rate of β-lipoprotein without changing its rate of synthesis or its distribution. Thus, although hepatic cholesterol synthesis can increase to compensate for loss, the new cholesterol need not appear as a constituent of β-lipoprotein, unless of course its synthesis was required to aid triglyceride transport. This suggests that it may be advantageous to administer at the same time as an acid-binding agent, an agent which reduces hepatic triglyceride synthesis or an agent which inhibits cholesterol biosynthesis before mevalonate is formed. Such combinations are being sought. Cholestyramine and nicotinic acid (Moutafis et al., 1971) and DEAE-Sephadex and clofibrate produce synergism in reduction of cholesterol levels (Howard and Hyams, 1971).

Neomycin, a basic antibiotic which is not absorbed, lowers cholesterol levels in man. As a result of its properties as a base, it induces marked precipitation of both fatty acids and bile acids within the intestinal lumen of healthy subjects (Thompson et al., 1971). N-Methylneomycin, which is basic but not an antibiotic, lowers plasma cholesterol and increases bile acid excretion in man and chicks (Van de Bosch and Claes, 1967).

5 Future trends

In the management of hyperlipidaemic patients, clinicians are now thinking in terms of correcting abnormal lipoprotein patterns. As lipid profile test kits become more readily available and it becomes possible to monitor lipoprotein patterns during treatment, the choice of diet, drug, or combination most likely to be effective will be placed on a firmer foundation. Undoubtedly, it will be found that a particular drug will not correct all examples of a particular abnormal pattern, and the possible biochemical defects responsible for that pattern will need to be considered. An attempt has been made here to summarize the biochemical actions of hypolipidaemic agents. Certain modes of action have been seen to be untenable for proposed therapeutic agents, but others appear to be acceptable and may provide a starting point for the design of hypolipidaemic agents having a specific mode of action.

References

Abdulla, Y. H. and Adams, C. W. M. (1971). *Atherosclerosis*, **13**, 61.

Achor, R. P. W., Winkelman, R. K. and Perry, H. O. (1961). *Proc. Staff Meet. Mayo Clin.* **36**, 217.

Arnold, A., Potts, G. O., McAuliff, J. P., Christiansen, R. G. and Miller, T. C. (1966). *Proc. Soc. Exp. Biol. Med.* **121**, 122.

Avigan, J., Steinberg, D., Vroman, H. E., Thompson, M. J. and Mosettig, E. (1960). *J. Biol. Chem.* **235**, 3123.

Azarnoff, D. L., Tucker, D. R. and Barr, G. A. (1965). *Metabolism*, **14**, 959.

Bach, F. L. (1970). In "Medicinal Chemistry" 3rd ed. (Ed. A. Burger), p. 1149. John Wiley, New York.

Bach, F. L., Barclay, J. C. and Cohen, E. (1967). *J. Med. Chem.* **10**, 802.

Bach, F. L., Barclay, J. C., Kende, F. and Cohen, E. (1968). *J. Med. Chem.* **11**, 987.

Baer, J. E., Russo, H. F., Brooks, A. V. and Beyer, K. H. (1959). *Pharmacologist*, **1**, 53

Barnhart, J. W., Johnson, J. D., Rytler, D. J. and Failey, R. B. (1972). *Advan. Exp. Med. Biol.* **26**, 275.

Barrett, A. M. (1966). *Brit. J. Pharmacol.* **26**, 363.

Barrett, A. M. and Thorp, J. M. (1968). *Brit. J. Pharmacol. Chemother.* **32**, 381.

Beaumont, J. L., Carlson, L. A., Cooper, G. R., Fejfar, Z., Fredrickson, D. S. and Strasser, T. (1970). *Bull. W.H.O.* **43**, 891.

Beckman, R., Hillman, G., Lagler, F., Lintz, W. and Vollenberg, W. (1972). *Advan. Exp. Med. Biol.* **26**, 276.

Beg, Z. H. and Lupien, P. J. (1972). *Biochim. Biophys. Acta*, **260**, 439.

Beher, W. T., Baker, G. D. and Anthony, W. L. (1957). *Circ. Res.* **5**, 202.

Best, M. M. and Duncan, C. H., (1964). *J. Lab. Clin. Med.* **64**, 634.

Best, M. M. and Duncan, C. H. (1970). *J. Atheroscler. Res.* **12**, 185.

Bhattathiry, E. P. M. and Siperstein, M. D. (1963). *J. Clin. Invest.* **42**, 1613.

Blank, B., Pfeiffer, F. R., Greenberg, C. M. and Kerwin, J. F. (1963). *J. Med. Chem.* **6**, 554.

Blank, B., Greenberg, C. M. and Kerwin, J. F. (1964). *J. Med. Chem.* **7**, 53.

Blank, B., Rice, E. G., Pfeiffer, F. R. and Greenberg, C. M. (1966). *J. Med. Chem.* **9**, 10.

Blohm, T. R. (1972). *Ann. Rep. Med. Chem.* **7**, 169.

Blohm, T. R. (1973). *Ann. Rep. Med. Chem.* **8**, 183.

Blohm, T. R., Kariya, T. and Laughlin, M. W. (1959). *Arch. Biochem. Biophys.* **85**, 250.

Burch, R. E. and Curran, G. L., (1969). *J. Lipid Res.* **10**, 668.

Carlson, L. A. (1960). *Acta Med. Scand.* **167**, 399.

Carlson, L. A. and Orö, L. (1962). *Acta Med. Scand.* **172**, 641.

Carlson, L. A., Hedbom, C., Helgstrand, E., Sjöberg, B. and Stjernström, N. E. (1969). *Adv. Exp. Med. Biol.* **4**, 85.

Carlson, L. A., Walldius, G. and Butcher, R. W. (1972). *Atherosclerosis*, **16**, 349.

Cook, R. P. and MacDougall, J. D. B. (1968). *Brit. J. Exp. Pathol.* **49**, 265.

The Coronary Drug Project Research Group (1970). *J. Amer. Med. Ass.* **214**, 1303.

The Coronary Drug Project Research Group (1972). *J. Amer. Med. Ass.* **220**, 996.

Cottet, J., Rede, J., Krumm-Heller, C. and Trichaud, M. E. (1953). *Bull. Acad. Nat. Med., Paris.* **137**, 441.

Counsell, R. E., Klimstra, P. D., Ranney, R. E. and Cook, D. L. (1962a). *J. Med. Pharm. Chem.* **5**, 720.

Counsell, R. E., Klimstra, P. D. and Ranney, R. E. (1962b). *J. Med. Pharm. Chem.* **5**, 1224.

Counsell, R. E., Klimstra, P. D., Nysted, L. N. and Ranney, R. E. (1965). *J. Med. Chem.* **8**, 45.

Craig, G. M. (1972). *Atherosclerosis,* **15**, 265.

Craig, G. M. and Walton, K. W. (1972). *Atherosclerosis,* **15**, 189.

Crombie, L. (1957). *Ann. Rep. Progr. Chem.* **54**, 207.

Ditschuneit, H., Ditschuneit, H. H., Klor, H. U., Rakow, D. and Schwandt, P. (1972). *Advan. Exp. Med. Biol.* **26**, 287.

Dujovne, C. A., Weiss, P. and Bianchine, J. R. (1971). *Clin. Pharmacol. Ther.* **12**, 117.

de Duve, C. and Baudhuin, P. (1966). *Physiol. Rev.* **46**, 323.

Dvornik, D. and Kraml, M. (1963). *Proc. Soc. Exp. Biol. Med.* **112**, 1012.

Dvornik, D., Kraml, M., Dubuc, J., Girner, M. and Gaudry, R. (1963). *J. Amer. Chem. Soc.* **85**, 3309.

Einarsson, K., Gustafsson, J-A. and Hellström, K. (1974). *Biochem. Pharmacol.* **23**, 13.

Eskelson, C. D., Cazee, C. R., Anthony, W., Towne, J. C. and Walske, B. R. (1970). *J. Med. Chem.* **13**, 215.

Fallon, H. J., Adams, L. L. and Lamb, R. G. (1971). *Lipids,* **7**, 106.

Figmonari, G. M. and Rodwell, V. W. (1965). *Science,* **147**, 1038.

Fisher, J. N. and Ball, E. G. (1967). *Biochemistry,* **6**, 637.

Fletscher, K. and Myant, N. B. (1958). *J. Physiol. (London),* **144**, 361.

Fletscher, K. and Myant, N. B. (1960). *J. Physiol. (London),* **154**, 145.

Fredrickson, D. S. and Steinberg, D. (1957). *Circulation,* **15**, 391.

Fredrickson, D. S., Levy, R. I. and Lees, R. S. (1967). *New England J. Med.* **276**, 94, 148, 215 and 273.

Fukushima, H., Aono, S., Nakamura, Y., Endo, M. and Imai, T. (1969). *J. Atherosclerosis Res.* **10**, 403.

Furman, R. H., Alaupovic, P. and Howard, R. P. (1967). *In* "Progress in Biochemical Pharmacology" (Eds D. Kritchevsky, R. Paoletti and D. Steinberg), vol. 2, p. 215. S. Karger, Basel.

Furman, R. H., Alaupovic, P., Bradford, R. H. and Howard, R. P. (1968). *In* "Progress in Biochemical Pharmacology" (Eds C. J. Miras, A. N. Howard and R. Paoletti), vol. 4, p. 334. S. Karger, Basel.

Gilfillan, J. L., Hunt, V. M. and Huff, J. W. (1971). *Proc. Soc. Exp. Biol.* **136**, 1274.

Giocoli, G., Tepperman, H. M. and Tepperman, J. (1971). *Proc. Soc. Exp. Biol. Med.* **138**, 512.

Glorr, U. and Wiss, O. (1959). *Arch. Biochem. Biophys.* **83**, 216.

Glueck, C. J. (1971). *Metabolism,* **20**, 691.

Goldstein, J. L. and Brown, M. S. (1973). *Proc. Nat. Acad. Sci.* **70**, 2166, 2804.

Goodman, D. S. and Noble, R. P. (1968). *J. Clin. Invest.* **47**, 231.

Gordon, S. and Cekleniak, W. P. (1968). *J. Med. Chem.* **11**, 993.

Gould, R. G. (1955). *Trans. N.Y. Acad. Sci.* **18**, 123, 129.

Gould, R. G. and Swyrd, E. A. (1966). *J. Lipid Res.* **7**, 698.

Greene, H. L., Herman, R. H. and Zakim, D. (1970). *Proc. Soc. Exp. Biol. Med.* **134**, 1035.

Gries, F. A., Miss, H. D., Canzler, H., Koschinsky, T., Vogelberg, K. H. and Jahnke, K. (1972). *Advan. Exp. Med. Biol.* **26**, 297.

Grisar, J. M., Parker, R. A., Kariya, T., Blohm, T. R., Fleming, R. W., Petrow, V., Wenstrup, D. L. and Johnson, R. G. (1972). *J. Med. Chem.* **15**, 1273.

Grundy, S. M., Ahrens Jr., E. H., Salen, G., Schreibman, P. H. and Nestel, P. J. (1972). *J. Lipid Res.* **13**, 531.

Guder, W., Nolte, I. and Wieland, O. (1968). *Eur. J. Biochem.* **4**, 271.

Hamilton, R. L. (1972). *Advan. Exp. Med. Biol.* **26**, 7.

Hamilton, J. G., Sullivan, A. C., Gutierrez, M. and Miller, O. N. (1971). *Fed. Proc.* **30**, 519.

Hansch, C. and Fujita, T. (1964). *J. Amer. Chem. Soc.* **86**, 1616.

Havel, R. J., Shore, V. G., Shore, B. and Bier, D. M. (1970). *Circ. Res.* **27**, 595.

Havel, R. J. and Kane, J. P. (1973). *Ann. Rev. Pharmacol.* **13**, 287.

Hazzard, W. R., Spiger, M. J., Bagdade, J. D. and Bierman, E. L. (1969). *New Eng. J. Med.* **280**, 471.

Hess, R. and Bencze, W. L. (1968). *Experientia*, **24**, 418.

Holmes, W. L. and DiTullio, N. W. (1962). *Amer. J. Clin. Nutr.* **10**, 310.

Howard, A. N. and Hyams, D. E. (1971). *Brit. Med. J.* **3**, 25.

Huff, J. W. and Gilfillan, J. L. (1960). *Proc. Soc. Exp. Biol. Med.* **103**, 41.

Hughes, G. M. K., Moore, P. F. and Stebbins, R. B. (1964). *J. Med. Chem.* **7**, 511.

Hughes, G. M. K. and Moore, P. F. (1967). *Ind. Chim. Belge*, **32**, 292.

Hulcher, F. H. (1971). *Arch. Biochem. Biophys.* **146**, 422.

Humber, L. G., Kraml, M. and Dubuc, J. (1962). *Biochem. Pharmacol.* **11**, 755.

Humber, L. G., Chappel, C. I., Marton, A. V., Kraml, M. and Dubuc, J. (1966). *J. Med. Chem.* **9**, 329.

Imai, T., Kikuchi, S., Matsuo, T., Suzuoki, Z. and Nishikawa, K. (1967). *Atherosclerosis Res.* **7**, 671.

Imai, Y., Matsumura, H., Tamura, S. and Shimamoto, K. (1973). *Atherosclerosis*, **17**, 131.

Jepson, E. M., Small, E., Grayson, M. F., Bance, G. and Billimoria, J. D. (1972). *Atherosclerosis*, **16**, 9.

Jouanneteau, J. and Zwingelstein, G. (1961). *Compt. Rend.* **252**, 1380.

Kariya, T., Blohm, T. R., Grizar, J. M., Parker, R. A. and Martin, J. R. (1972). *Advan. Exp. Med. Biol.* **26**, 302.

Katterman, R., Arnold, R. and Creutzfeldt, W. (1972). *Arzneim.-Forsch.* **22**, 616.

Kelly, L. A. and Ho, R. S. (1968). *Fed Proc.* **27**, 242.

Kirschner, K., Henning, U. and Lynen, F. (1961). *Ann. Chem. Liebig's*, **644**, 48.

Kohen, F., Ranade, V. V. and Counsell, R. E. (1972). *J. Med. Chem.* **15**, 1129.

Kritchevsky, D. (1964). *Metabolism*, **9**, 984.

Kritchevsky, D. (1971). *In* "Metabolic Effects of Nicotinic Acid and its Derivatives" (Eds K. F. Gey and L. A. Carlson), p. 541.

Kritchevsky, D. and Tepper, S. A. (1962). *Arch. Int. Pharmacodyn. Ther.* **138**, 349.

Kritchevsky, D. and Tepper, S. A. (1969). *Experientia*, **25**, 699.

Kritchevsky, D. and Tepper, S. A. (1971). *Arzneim.-Forsch.* **21**, 1024.

Kritchevsky, D. and Tepper, S. A. (1972). *Proc. Soc. Exp. Biol. Med.* **139**, 1284.
Kritchevsky, D. and Tepper, S. A. (1973). *Arzneim.-Forsch.* **23**, 858.
Kritchevsky, D., Tepper, S. A., Sallata, P., Kabakjian, J. R. and Cristofalo, V. J. (1969). *Proc. Soc. Exp. Biol. Med.* **132**, 76.
Kupiecki, F. and Marshall, N. B. (1968). *J. Pharmacol. Exp. Ther.* **160**, 166.
Lack, L. and Weiner, I. M. (1963). *J. Pharmacol. Exptl. Ther.* **139**, 248.
Lamb, R. G. and Fallon, H. J. (1972). *J. Biol Chem.* **247**, 1281.
Lamb, R. G., Hill, P. M. and Fallon, H. J. (1973). *J. Lipid Res.* **14**, 459.
LaRosa, J. C., Levy, R. I., Herbert, P., Lux, S. E. and Fredrickson, D. S. (1970). *Biochem. Biophys. Res. Commun.* **41**, 57.
Lewis, B. (1973). *J. Clin. Pathol.* **26** *suppl.* (Ass. Clin. Path.) **5**, 26.
Levy, R. I. and Rifkind, B. M. (1973). *Drugs*, **6**, 12.
Levy, R. I., Fredrickson, D. S., Shulman, R., Biheimer, D. W., Breslow, J. L., Stone, N. J., Lux, S. E., Sloan, H. R., Krauss, R. M. and Herbert, P. N. (1972). *Ann. Intern. Med.* **77**, 267.
Lupien, P. J., Brun, D. and Moorjani, S. (1973a). *Lancet*, 1256.
Lupien, P. J., Tremblay, M. and Beg, Z. H. (1973b). *Atherosclerosis*, **18**, 407.
Maragoudakis, M. E. (1969). *J. Biol. Chem.* **244**, 5005.
Maragoudakis, M. E. (1970). *Biochemistry*, **9**, 413.
Maragoudakis, M. E., Harkin, H. and Wasvary, J. M. (1972). *J. Biol. Chem.* **247**, 342.
Merola, A. J. and Arnold, A. (1964). *Science*, **144**, 301.
Miettinen, T. A. (1968). *Clin. Chim. Acta*, **20**, 43.
Miettinen, T. A. (1972). *Atherosclerosis*, **15**, 163.
Mitropoulos, K. A. and Myant, N. B. (1965). *Biochem. J.* **94**, 594.
Morand, P., Bagli, J. F., Kraml, M. and Dubuc, J. (1964). *J. Med. Chem.* **7**, 504.
Morgan, J. P., Bianchine, J. R., Hsu, T. H. and Margolis, S. (1971). *Clin. Pharmacol. Ther.* **12**, 517.
Mosbach, E. H. (1969). *Adv. Exp. Med. Biol.* **4**, 421.
Moutafis, C. D. and Myant, N. B. (1969). *Clin. Sci.* **37**, 443.
Moutafis, C. D., Myant, N. B., Mancini, M. and Oriente, P. (1971). *Atherosclerosis*, **14**, 247.
Mukherjee, S. and Bhose, A. (1968). *Biochim. Biophys. Acta*, **164**, 357.
Nakamura, K., Toyota, A., Masuda, Y. and Nakamura, H. (1967). *J. Atherosclerosis Res.* **7**, 783.
Nash, D. T. (1972). *Advan. Exp. Med. Biol.* **26**, 311.
Nestel, P. J. and Austin, W. (1968). *J. Atherosclerosis Res.* **8**, 827.
Niemiro, R. and Fumagalli, R. (1965). *Biochim. Biophys. Acta*, **98**, 624.
Nikkila, E. A. and Kekki, M. (1972). *Eur. J. Clin. Invest.* **2**, 231.
Page, I. H. and Schneckloth, R. E. (1959). *Circulation,* **20**, 1075.
Parkinson, T. M., Gundersen, K. and Nelson, N. A. (1970). *Atherosclerosis*, **11**, 531.
Parsons, W. B. (1972). *Circulation*, **46**, Suppl. II, Abs. 60.
Pereira, J. N., Holland, G. F., Hochstein, F. A., Gilgore, S., Defelice, S. and Pinson, R. (1968). *J. Pharmacol. Exp. Ther.* **162**, 148.
Piccinini, F. (1962). *Arch. Ital. Sci. Farmacol.* **12**, 111.
Platt, D. S. and Cockrill, B. L. (1966). *Biochem. Pharmacol.* **15**, 927.
Platt, D. S. and Thorp, J. M. (1966). *Biochem. Pharmacol.* **15**, 915.
Polachek, A. A., Hatz, H. M. and Littman, M. (1972). *Advan. Exp. Med. Biol.* **26**, 316.
Popjak, G. (1959). *Tetrahedron Lett.* No. 19, p. 19.

Popjak, G., Cornforth, R. H. and Clifford, K. (1960). *Lancet*, **i**, 1270.

Ranade, V. V., Kohen, F. and Counsell, R. E. (1971). *J. Med. Chem.* **14**, 38.

Ranney, R. E. and Counsell, R. E. (1962). *Proc. Soc. Exp. Biol. Med.* **109**, 820.

Reddy, J., Svoboda, D. and Azarnoff, D. (1973). *Biochem. Biophys. Res. Commun.* **52**, 537.

Rodney, G., Black, M. L. and Bird, O. D. (1965). *Biochem. Pharmacol.* **14**, 445.

Roux, C. and Aubry, M. (1966). *C. R. Soc. Biol.* **160**, 1353.

Russo, C. and Mendlowitz, M. (1971). *Clin. Pharmacol. Ther.* **12**, 676.

Sachs, B. A. and Wolfman, L. (1962). *Circulation*, **26**, 669.

Scanu, A. M. and Wisdom, C. (1972). *Ann. Rev. Biochem.* **41**, 703.

Schacht, U. and Granzer, E. (1970). *Biochem. Pharmacol.* **19**, 2963.

Short, J. H., Biermacher, U., Dunnigan, D. A., Lambert, G. F., Martin, D. L., Nordeen, C. W. and Wright, H. B. (1965). *J. Med. Chem.* **8**, 223.

Singer, F. M., Januska, J. P. and Borman, A. (1959). *Proc. Soc. Exp. Biol. Med.* **102**, 370.

Siperstein, M. D. and Fagan, V. M. (1964). *Advan. Enzyme Regul.* **2**, 249.

Sirtori, C., Hurwitz, A., Sabih, K. and Azarnoff, D. L. (1971). *Lipids*, **7**, 96.

Skidmore, I. F., Schoenhaefer, P. S. and Kritchevsky, D. (1971). *Pharmacology*, **6**, 330.

Solberg, H. E., Aas, M. and Daae, L. N. W. (1972). *Biochim. Biophys. Acta*, **280**, 434.

Spector, A. A. and Soboroff, J. M. (1971). *Clin. Res.* **19**, 681.

Steinberg, D., Avigan, J. and Feigelson, E. B. (1961). *J. Clin. Invest.* **40**, 884.

Strisower, E. H., Nichols, A. V., Lindgren, F. T. and Smith L. (1965). *J. Lab. Clin. Med.* **65**, 748.

Tavormina, P. A. and Gibbs, M. (1957). *J. Amer. Chem. Soc.* **79**, 758.

Thompson, G. R., Barrowman, J., Gutierrez, L. and Dowling, R. H. (1971). *J. Clin. Invest.* **50**, 319.

Thorp, J. M. (1963). *J. Atheroscler. Res.* **3**, 351.

Thorp, J. M. (1970). Atherosclerosis: Proceedings of the Second International Symposium (Ed. R. J. Jones), p. 541. Springer-Verlag, Berlin, Heidelberg, New York.

Thorp, J. M. (1971). Proceedings, XIII Meeting of the European Society for the Study of Drug Toxicity, 98.

Thorp, J. M. (1973). Personal communication.

Timms, A. R., Griot, R. F. and Spirito, J. A. (1968). *Fed. Proc.* **27**, 242.

Timms, A. R., Kelly, L. A., Ho, R. S. and Trapold, J. H. (1969). *Biochem. Pharmacol.* **18**, 1861.

Tolman, E. L., Tepperman, H. M. and Tepperman, J. (1970). *Amer. J. Physiol.* **218**, 1313.

US Public Health Service Publication No. 1695 (1967).

Van den Bosch, J. F. and Claes, P. J. (1967). *In* "Progress in Biochemical Pharmacology" (Eds D. Kritchevsky, R. Paoletti and D. Steinberg), vol. 2, p. 97. S. Karger, Basel.

Venton, D. L., Kohen, F. and Counsell, R. E. (1973). *J. Med. Chem.* **16**, 571.

Walsh, M. R., Teal, S. W. and Gamble, W. (1969). *Arch. Biochem. Biophys.* **130**, 7.

Walton, K. W. and Williamson, N. (1968). *J. Atheroscler. Res.* **8**, 599.

Weber, G., Convery, H. J. H., Lea, M. A. and Stamm, N. B. (1966). *Science*, **154**, 1357.

Westerfeld, W. W., Richert, D. A. and Ruegamer, W. R. (1968). *Biochem. Pharmacol.* **17**, 1003.
Whayne, T. F. and Witiak, D. T. (1973). *J. Med. Chem.* **16**, 228.
White, L. W. (1971). *J. Pharmacol. Exp. Therap.* **178**, 361.
White, L. W. (1972). *Circ. Res.* **31**, 899.
Witiak, D. T., Feller, D. R., Stratford, E. S., Hackney, R. E. Nazareth, R. and Wagner, G. (1971a). *J. Med. Chem.* **14**, 754.
Witiak, D. T., Parker, R. A., Dempsey, M. E. and Ritter, M. C. (1971b). *J. Med. Chem.* **14**, 684.
Zakin, D., Paradini, R. S. and Herman, R. H. (1970). *Biochem. Pharmacol.* **19**, 305.
Zöllner, N., and Gudenzi, M. (1967). *In* "Progress in Biochemical Pharmacology" (Eds D. Kritchevsky, R. Paoletti and D. Steinberg), vol. 2, p. 406. S. Karger, Basel.

Laboratory Models for Atherosclerosis[1]

DAVID KRITCHEVSKY, BS, MS, PhD

The Wistar Institute of Anatomy and Biology, Philadelphia, Pennsylvania, USA

Atherosclerosis in man is a complex disease of multiple etiology, with numerous augmenting factors; it is a life-long process. Generally, no clinical episodes are observed until the disease is relatively far advanced. One of the challenges to research in this field has been to establish an animal model in which it would be possible to duplicate lesions of the type usually seen in man and to obtain those lesions in a short time while subjecting the animal to a minimum of physiological trauma. Such a model could then be subjected to studies involving those factors known to play a role in human atherosclerosis in efforts to arrest or reverse the disease. Several excellent reviews of this subject are available (Clarkson, 1963; Kritchevsky, 1964; Constantinides, 1965; Roberts and Straus, 1965).

Whatever modality is used to establish atherosclerosis, the disease in animals is almost always accompanied by hyperbetalipoproteinemia. Generally, ease of establishment of atherosclerosis is not so much a function of an animal's endogenous cholesterol level as it is of the animal's β-lipoprotein level. Table 1 presents data for some of the animal species used in atherosclerosis research.

This discussion will concern itself with the characteristics of the various species used in atherosclerosis research.

1 Dogs

When dogs were fed cholesterol for long periods of time they responded with hyperlipidemia but atherosclerosis was not observed (Shull and Mann,

[1] Supported, in part, by grants HE 03299 and HE 05209, and a research career award HL 0734 from the National Heart and Lung Institute, Bethesda, Maryland, USA.

TABLE 1

Species differences in serum lipids[a]

Species	Serum cholesterol (mg dl^{-1})	α Lipoprotein (mg dl^{-1})	β Lipoprotein (mg dl^{-1})	α/β
Cat	140	700	70	10·0
Dog	100	300	50	6·0
Chicken	100	100	160	0·6
Rat	80	150	80	1·9
Rabbit	50	100	100	1·0

[a] After Olson (1958).

1957). However, when thiouracil was added to the cholesterol-containing diet, lesions were observed (Steiner and Kendal, 1946; Steiner et al., 1949). The addition of butter to the cholesterol-thiouracil diet hastened the appearance of atheromatous lesions (DiLuzio and O'Neal, 1962). More recently Malmros and Sternby (1968) have shown that dogs fed a semi-synthetic diet containing a large (15–20 per cent) quantity of hydrogenated coconut oil and 5 per cent cholesterol will become atherosclerotic. While the diet may be extreme, it is more physiological than a regimen which requires chemical thyroidectomy.

2   Rats

The rat is considered to be a "resistant" species. This means that, although lesions can be induced by heroic means, the methodology does not lend itself to simple experimentation. Page and Brown (1952) maintained rats on cholesterol plus cholic acid and observed cholesteremia and aortic sudanophilia but no intimal changes.

Diets containing fat, cholesterol, cholic acid and thiouracil produced atherosclerosis in the rat (Hartroft et al., 1952; Malinow et al., 1954). When the dietary fat was saturated, thrombosis occurred, whereas peanut oil led to atherosclerosis (Gresham and Howard, 1960; 1961). Attempts to make these diets less toxic (by removal of the thiouracil) have led to formulation of diets high in butter, cholic acid and cholesterol (O'Neal et al., 1961; Still and O'Neal, 1962) or diets high in lard and cholesterol (Jones et al., 1957) which have elicited some aortic lesion. Thomas et al. (1965) have published details of a "standard" atherogenic rat diet.

Coronary atherosclerosis was induced in rats by feeding cholesterol to hypophysectomized rats (Patek *et al.*, 1963) or by feeding coconut oil to essential fatty acid-deficient animals (Morin *et al.*, 1964). Altschul (1950) attempted to induce atherosclerosis in other rodents by feeding cholesterol and found the gerbil and prairie gopher were resistant and the hamster, guinea pig and squirrel gave equivocal results. Only in the scorbutic guinea pig could atheromata be induced by a cholesterol-rich diet.

3 Chickens

Atherosclerosis can be induced in chickens by feeding cholesterol, undernutrition, stilbesterol administration, induction of hypertension and pancreatectomy (Katz and Stamler, 1953). Increasing levels of dietary cholesterol gave more severe lesions in a shorter period of time, but even 0·5 per cent cholesterol caused lesions to appear in 10 weeks in 80 per cent of the birds fed. Stamler *et al.* (1959) (Table 2) demonstrated that saturated fat or free fatty acids were more atherogenic than were unsaturated fats.

TABLE 2

Effect of fats (10 per cent) on cholesterol level and atherosclerosis in chickens fed 1 per cent cholesterol[a]

Fat	Plasma cholesterol (mg dl^{-1})	Atherosclerosis	
		Incidence (%)	Grade
Coconut oil	832	100	1·0
Olive oil	704	78	1·6
Oleic acid	839	11	0·5
Cottonseed oil	1252	90	1·4
Safflower oil	650	70	1·0
Linoleic acid	1528	100	1·4

[a] After Stamler *et al.* (1959).

4 Pigeons

The White Carneau pigeon develops spontaneous atherosclerotic lesions that resemble those seen in man (Lofland and Clarkson, 1959; Clarkson *et al.*, 1959a). Their serum cholesterol levels, however, are no higher than those of other pigeon strains that are free of atherosclerosis—suggesting genetic and/or metabolic factors (Table 3). Feeding of cholesterol to the White Carneau pigeon greatly increased the incidence and severity of the atherosclerotic lesion (Clarkson and Lofland, 1961). The severity and

TABLE 3
Spontaneous atherosclerosis in pigeons[a]

Breed	Age (years)	Sex	Number	Serum cholesterol (mg dl^{-1})	Aortic area (%) with athero-sclerosis
Racing Homer	4·4	M	10	361	0·5
		F	3	303	0·0
Show Racer	6·8	M	7	364	1·5
		F	7	318	1·2
Silver King	7·4	M	12	328	12·0
		F	12	430	11·0
White Carneau	7·8	M	12	372	9·3
		F	13	383	13·2

[a] After Lofland and Clarkson (1959).

extent of lesions in the White Carneau pigeon were also affected by the type of fat (saturated > unsaturated) and the level of dietary protein (30 per cent > 15 per cent) (Lofland et al., 1961). These findings suggest that interaction of all dietary components is important in determining the effect of any one of them.

5 Pigs

The pig is susceptible to spontaneous atherosclerosis but more severe lesions can be induced by feeding a high fat, high cholesterol diet. The advantages of using swine are the facts that the pig is an omnivore, his lesions resemble those of man and he is large enough to permit surgical manipulation. The disadvantages of this model include the expense of feeding and otherwise maintaining pigs. Gottlieb and Lalich (1954) and Skold and Getty (1961) documented the increasing levels of spontaneous atherosclerosis observed in ageing pigs (Table 4). Rowsell et al. (1958; 1960) found that both cholesteremia and atherosclerosis were enhanced by saturated fat and cholesterol. Downie et al. (1963) found that the most severe atheromatosis was induced by diets containing lard and cholesterol (Table 5).

Calloway and Potts (1962) produced atherosclerosis in pigs using a diet low in protein and high in saturated fat.

TABLE 4

Spontaneous atherosclerosis in swine[a]

Age (years)	Sex	Number of aortas examined	Sclerotic aortas Number (%)
0·3–0·7	M/F	493	16 (3)
1–2	F	676	91 (13)
2–3	F	362	92 (25)
2–3	M	28	7 (25)
3+	F	69	21 (30)
3+	M	147	51 (35)

[a] After Gottlieb and Lalich (1954).

TABLE 5

Dietary induction of atherosclerosis in swine[a]

Diet	Serum cholesterol (mg dl^{-1})	Serum lipoproteins (mg dl^{-1}) S_f0–20	20–400	Aortic lesions (%)
Control	115	133	4	16
25% lard	135	144	4	22
25% egg yolk	158	220	13	33
25% lard/cholesterol	236	401	34	42

[a] After Downie et al. (1963).

6 Rabbits

Probably the animal most widely used to date in atherosclerosis research has been the rabbit. The rabbit is readily available, easy to feed and handle, is large enough for tissue and blood studies and can be rendered atherosclerotic quickly and easily. On the debit side are the facts that the rabbit is normally a vegetarian and that the lesions are neither constituted nor distributed as they are in man. Nevertheless, this species has borne the brunt of the research onslaught over the sixty odd years since Saltykow (1908) and Ignatowski (1909) found that diets rich in milk, meat and eggs produced atherosclerosis in the rabbit's aorta. It was later shown by Anitschkow (1913) and others (Wesselkin, 1913; Wacker and Hueck, 1913; Anitschkow and Chalatow, 1913) that cholesterol was the atherogenic factor in the early diets.

The amount of cholesterol and amount and type of fat in the diet affect the severity of the observed lesions. Scebat *et al.* (1961) showed that low levels of dietary cholesterol, if fed for sufficiently long periods, produced atheromata of a level of severity similar to that observed on regimens higher in cholesterol (Table 6). We have devoted many years to

TABLE 6

Response of rabbits to different dosages of cholesterol[a]

Feeding period (days)	Daily dose (mg)					
	250		500		1000	
	SC[b]	Atheroma	SC	Atheroma	SC	Atheroma
30	271	0·9	651	1·3	813	1·8
90	250	–	1152	2·3	1072	3·0
130	545	3·0	1103	3·3	1095	3·8

[a] After Scebat *et al.* (1961).
[b] Serum cholesterol (mg dl^{-1}).

the investigation of the effect of the fatty vehicle on experimental atherosclerosis (summarized by Kritchevsky, 1970) and have found that the severity of atherosclerosis is inversely proportional to the iodine value of the fat (Table 7). In addition, it has been observed that cholesterol fed

TABLE 7

Effect of fat on experimental atherosclerosis in rabbits[a]
(2 per cent cholesterol; 6 per cent fat. Two month feeding)

Fat	Iodine value	Survival	Serum cholesterol (mg dl^{-1})	Average atheromata	
				Arch	Thoracic
No fat	–	10/14	1214	3·1	2·3
Coconut oil	10	12/14	2827	3·1	2·5
Lard	66	9/14	2245	2·7	2·0
Hydrogenated corn oil	79	13/14	1984	2·5	1·7
Corn oil	134	13/14	1908	1·6	1·3

[a] After Kritchevsky (1970).

in the absence of other fat or in the presence of fat plus free fatty acid is no more cholesteremic than a cholesterol-fat diet, but much more atherogenic.

Lesions begin to appear after two weeks on a cholesterol-no-fat or cholesterol-fatty acid diet, but on the cholesterol-corn oil diet lesions are generally not seen until after four weeks of feeding (Kritchevsky and Tepper, 1973).

Among the dietary fats, peanut oil is remarkable because this fat, when fed with cholesterol, is almost as atherogenic as coconut oil (Kritchevsky *et al.*, 1971a). However, chemical randomization of this oil renders it significantly less atherogenic (Kritchevsky *et al.*, 1973b) (Table 8).

TABLE 8

Influence of various fats on atherosclerosis in rabbits[a]
(2 per cent cholesterol; 6 per cent fat. Fed 60 days)

Fat	Survival ratio	Serum cholesterol (mg dl^{-1})	Atherosclerosis ± SEM	
			Arch	Thoracic
Series I (5 experiments)				
Coconut oil (CNO)	55/58	1397	2·06 ± 0·14	1·55 ± 0·12
Peanut oil (PNO)	54/58	1302	1·94 ± 0·14	1·25 ± 0·11
Corn oil (CO)	55/58	1479	1·57 ± 0·14	1·03 ± 0·09
Series II (3 experiments)				
Peanut oil	27/31	1873	2·22 ± 0·15[b]	1·54 ± 0·14[c]
Randomized peanut oil	31/31	1833	1·31 ± 0·12	1·05 ± 0·10
Corn oil	28/31	1678	1·18 ± 0·12	0·95 ± 0·12

[a] After Kritchevsky *et al.* (1971; 1973b).
[b] PNO versus randomized PNO or CO, $p < 0.001$.
[c] PNO versus randomized PNO or CO, $p < 0.01$.

Lambert *et al.* (1958) and Malmros and Wigand (1959; 1960) showed that a semi-synthetic diet high in saturated fat was sufficient to cause hyperbetalipoproteinemia and hypercholesteremia in the rabbit. Kritchevsky and Tepper (1968) and Kritchevsky *et al.* (1968a; 1973c) have since shown that the type of carbohydrate present in the semi-synthetic diet affects the severity of the atherosclerosis (sucrose being more atherogenic than glucose, for instance) and the addition of hydrogenated coconut oil to laboratory chow does not render it atherogenic, suggesting a "protective" factor in the chow—possibly the non-nutritive fiber. Peanut oil is not atherogenic when present in the semi-synthetic, cholesterol-free diet, suggesting that it is not atherogenic *per se*, but rather that, somehow, it is synergistic with dietary cholesterol (Kritchevsky, unpublished observation).

The cholesterol-induced rabbit lesion generally becomes more severe

with time even after cessation of cholesterol feeding. Addition of unsaturated fat to the diet after cholesterol has been removed inhibits to
some degree the exacerbation of the lesions (Kritchevsky and Tepper,
1962; Vles et al., 1964).

It is possible to use the cholesterol-fed rabbit as a model to test the
effects of hypocholesteremic (and presumably anti-atherogenic) drugs.
Table 9 summarizes some experiments of this type.

TABLE 9

Influence of drugs on experimental atherosclerosis in rabbits

Drug	Number	Serum cholesterol (mg dl^{-1})	Atheromata		Reference
			Arch	Thoracic	
DT$_4$ (0·5–1 mg)	29	1372	1·78[a]	1·34	Kritchevsky et al.
Control	33	1913	2·76	1·90	(1961)
Linolexamide (0·1%)	22	1115	1·10[a]	0·66	Kritchevsky and
Control	19	1968	1·86	0·91	Tepper (1967)
Atromid-S (0·3%)	42	1851	1·90[a]	1·29	Kritchevsky et al.
Control	41	1996	2·29	1·38	(1968b)
DH 581 (1%)	28	1283	1.57[a]	0·98[a]	Kritchevsky et al.
Control	29	1889	2·05	1·38	(1971b)
Colestipol	30	1727	1·36[a]	0·97[a]	Kritchevsky et al.
Control	29	1889	1·88	1·31	(1973a)

    [a] Significantly different from control.
DT$_4$ = D-Thyroxine.
Linolexamide = N-Cyclohexyl-linoleamide.
Atromid-S = Ethyl p-chlorophenoxyisobutyrate.
DH 581 = 4,4'-(Isopropylidenedithio)bis-(2,6-di-t-butylphenol).
Colestipol = Tetraethylenepentamine-epichlorhydrin copolymer.

7   Non-human primates

Currently the trend in atherosclerosis research has swung toward use of
monkeys or baboons with good reason. Except for being expensive to
purchase and maintain and hard to handle, the monkey is an omnivore,
shows a progression of lesions similar to those seen in man and has a
distribution of lesions similar to that observed in humans.

However, all species of monkey do not react similarly to the same
dietary stimulus. The rhesus monkey (Macaca mulatta) responded to
pyridoxine deficiency by developing arteriosclerosis (Rinehart and
Greenberg, 1949). The rhesus monkey was also made atherosclerotic by

feeding cholesterol. The lesions appeared to be related to the degree and severity of hypercholesteremia and myocardial infarction has been observed (Taylor *et al.*, 1962; 1963). Atherosclerotic plaques have also been observed in cebus monkeys (*Cebus fatuella*) maintained on diets high in cholesterol and low in sulfur amino acids (Mann *et al.*, 1953).

In a survey of serum cholesterol levels and spontaneous atherosclerosis in New World monkeys, Lofland *et al.* (1967) found relatively little variation in cholesterol levels but large differences in degree of atherosclerosis (Table 10).

TABLE 10

Serum lipids and spontaneous atherosclerosis in monkeys[a]

Species	Number	Cholesterol (mg dl^{-1})		Atherosclerotic index (% Sudanophilia)
		Total	β-Lipoprotein	
Squirrel (*Saimiri scuireus*)	220	105	74	7·6
Capuchin (*Cebus apella*)	21	98	76	0·0
Ringtail (*Cebus albifrons*)	57	90	67	2·8
Spider (*Ateles*)	29	130	118	2·5
Woolly (*Lagothrix lagothrix*)	20	133	118	1·0

[a] After Lofland *et al.* (1967).

Cebus monkeys (*Cebus albifrons*) were made atherosclerotic by feeding cholesterol and coconut oil or butter (Wissler *et al.*, 1962) but cholesterol plus lard seemed to be without effect (MacNintch *et al.*, 1967). Portman and Andrus (1965) fed three species of monkey 0·5 per cent cholesterol and coconut or corn oil (Table 11) and found variable effects on cholesteremia and atherosclerosis. Squirrel monkeys (*Saimiri sciureus*) fed a cholesterol-high protein diet exhibited more severe atherosclerosis than did monkeys fed a cholesterol-low protein regimen (Middleton *et al.*, 1967).

It is possible to induce atherosclerosis in baboons by feeding cholesterol-containing diets (Gillman and Gilbert, 1957; Gresham *et al.*, 1965). Strong and McGill (1967) observed relatively severe aortic sudanophilia in baboons fed a high cholesterol-low protein-saturated fat diet.

We (Kritchevsky *et al.*, 1974) have fed baboons a semi-synthetic diet

TABLE 11

Diet and atherosclerosis in three species of monkeys[a]

	Species					
	Cebus		Woolly		Squirrel	
	SC[b]	A[c]	SC	A	SC	A
Control	157	0·0	239	2·1	207	17·5
Corn oil + cholesterol (0·5%)	344	0·2	358	19·7	314	13·0
Coconut oil + cholesterol (0·5%)	366	0·01	623	24·8	419	56·3

[a] After Portman and Andrus (1965).
[b] SC—Serum cholesterol (mg dl^{-1}).
[c] A—Per cent surface with sudanophilia.

(25 per cent casein, 40 per cent carbohydrate, 14 per cent hydrogenated coconut oil) for one year and observed sudanophilia of varying severity based upon the type of carbohydrate in the diet. The results are summarized in Table 12. Experiments with labelled cholesterol and its

TABLE 12

Diet[a] and aortic sudanophilia in baboons

	Serum lipids (mg dl^{-1}) ± SEM		Aortic
Carbohydrate	Triglyceride (75)[b]	Cholesterol (121)[b]	sudanophilia (%)
Fructose	129 ± 11	162 ± 10	11·2 ± 5·7
Sucrose	116 ± 8	152 ± 9	6·7 ± 4·7
Starch	108 ± 5	156 ± 8	9·3 ± 4.3
Glucose	105 ± 7	151 ± 11	6·2 ± 4·8
Control	78 ± 4	113 ± 3	0·02 ± 0·02

After Kritchevsky et al. (1974).
[a] 40 per cent carbohydrate; 25 per cent casein; 14 per cent hydrogenated coconut oil; fed 12 months.
[b] (Number) = starting average for all animals.

precursors suggest that reduced synthesis of bile acids may be one factor contributing towards the hypercholesteremia observed on these cholesterol-free diets.

The search for a suitable animal model and a suitable means of induction of atherosclerosis continues. To date, the major emphasis has been on dietary induction of atherosclerosis but the ideal model must be an animal that reacts to other risk factors (e.g. hypertension, stress) as man does.

The perfect model will be one in which atherosclerosis can be produced by an interaction of factors and treated successfully by drugs, diet or some other modality in a manner that is readily adapted to the human.

References

Altschul, R. (1950). "Selected Studies on Arteriosclerosis". C. C. Thomas, Springfield, Illinois.

Anitschkow, N. (1913). *Beitr. Pathol. Anat. Allg. Pathol.* **56**, 379.

Anitschkow, N. and Chalatow, S. (1913). *Zentralbl. Allg. Pathol. Pathol. Anat.* **24**, 1.

Calloway, D. H. and Potts, R. B. (1962). *Cir. Res.* **11**, 47.

Clarkson, T. B. (1963). *In* "Advances in Lipid Research" (Eds R. Paoletti and D. Kritchevsky), vol. 1, p. 211. Academic Press, New York and London.

Clarkson, T. B. and Lofland, H. B. (1961). *Circ. Res.* **9**, 106.

Clarkson, T. B., Prichard, R. W., Netsky, M. G. and Lofland, H. B. (1959). *Arch. Pathol.* 143.

Constandinides, P. (1965). "Experimental Atherosclerosis", vol. 68, p. 143. Elsevier, Amsterdam.

DiLuzio, N. R. and O'Neal, R. M. (1962). *Exp. Mol. Pathol.* **1**, 122.

Downie, H. G., Mustard, J. F. and Rowsell, H. C. (1963). *Ann. N.Y. Acad. Sci.* **104**, 539.

Gillman, J. and Gilbert, C. (1957). *Exp. Med. Surg.* **15**, 181.

Gottlieb, H. and Lalich, J. J. (1954). *Amer. J. Pathol.* **30**, 851.

Gresham, G. A. and Howard, A. N. (1960). *Brit. J. Exp. Pathol.* **41**, 395.

Gresham, G. A. and Howard, A. N. (1961). *Brit. J. Exp. Pathol.* **42**, 166.

Gresham, G. A., Howard, A. N., McQueen, J. and Bowyer, D. E. (1965). *Brit. J. Exp. Pathol.* **46**, 94.

Hartroft, W. S., Ridout, J. H., Sellars, E. A. and Best, C. H. (1952). *Proc. Soc. Exp. Biol. Med.* **81**, 384.

Ignatowski, A. (1909). *Arch. Pathol. Anat. Physiol.* **198**, 248.

Jones, R. J., Wissler, R. W. and Huffman, S. (1957). *Arch. Pathol.* **63**, 593.

Katz, L. N. and Stamler, J. (1953). "Experimental Atherosclerosis". C. C. Thomas, Springfield, Illinois.

Kritchevsky, D. (1964). *In* "Lipid Pharmacology" (Ed. R. Paoletti), p. 63. Academic Press, New York and London.

Kritchevsky, D. (1970). *Amer. J. Clin. Nutr.* **23**, 1105.

Kritchevsky, D. and Tepper, S. A. (1962). *J. Atheroscler. Res.* **2**, 471.

Kritchevsky, D. and Tepper, S. A. (1967). *J. Atheroscler. Res.* **7**, 527.

Kritchevsky, D. and Tepper, S. A. (1968). *J. Atheroscler. Res.* **8**, 357.

Kritchevsky, D. and Tepper, S. A. (1973). *Nutr. Reports Int.* **8**, 163.

Kritchevsky, D., Moynihan, J. L., Langan, J., Tepper, S. A. and Sachs, M. L. (1961). *J. Atheroscler. Res.* **1**, 211.

Kritchevsky, D., Sallata, P. and Tepper, S. A. (1968a). *J. Atheroscler. Res.* **8**, 697.

Kritchevsky, D., Sallata, P. and Tepper, S. A. (1968b). *J. Atheroscler. Res.* **8**, 755.

Kritchevsky, D., Kim, H. K. and Tepper, S. A. (1971a). *Proc. Soc. Exp. Biol. Med.* **136**, 1216.

Kritchevsky, D., Tepper, S. A., Vesselinovitch, D. and Wissler, R. W. (1971b). *Atherosclerosis*, **14**, 53.

Kritchevsky, D., Kim, H. K. and Tepper, S. A. (1973a). *Proc. Soc. Exp. Biol. Med.* **142**, 185.

Kritchevsky, D., Tepper, S. A., Vesselinovitch, D. and Wissler, R. W. (1973b). *Atherosclerosis*, **17**, 225.

Kritchevsky, D., Tepper, S. A. and Kitagawa, M. (1973c). *Nutr. Reports Int.* **7**, 193.

Kritchevsky, D., Davidson, L. M., Shapiro, I. L., Kim, H. K., Kitagawa, M., Malhotra, S., Nair, P. P., Clarkson, T. B., Bersohn, I. and Winter, P. A. D. (1974). *Amer. J. Clin. Nutr.* **27**, 29.

Lambert, G. F., Miller, J. P., Olsen, R. T. and Frost, D. V. (1958). *Proc. Soc. Exp. Biol. Med.* **97**, 544.

Lofland, H. B. and Clarkson, T. B. (1959). *Circ. Res.* **7**, 234.

Lofland, H. B., Clarkson, T. B. and Goodman, H. O. (1961). *Circ. Res.* **9**, 919.

Lofland, H. B., St. Clair, R. W., MacNintch, J. E. and Prichard, R. W. (1967). *Arch. Pathol.* **83**, 211.

MacNintch, J. E., St. Clair, R. W., Lehner, N. D. M., Clarkson, T. B. and Lofland, H. B. (1967). *Lab. Invest.* **16**, 444.

Malinow, M. R., Hojman, D. and Pellegrino, A. (1954). *Acta Cardiol.* **5**, 480.

Mann, G. V., Andrus, S. B., McNally, A. and Stare, F. J. (1953). *J. Exp. Med.* **98**, 195.

Malmros, H. and Sternby, N. H. (1968). *In* "Progress in Biochemical Pharmacology" (Eds C. J. Meras, A. N. Howard and R. Paoletti), vol. 4, p. 482. S. Karger, Basel.

Malmros, H. and Wigand, G. (1959). *Lancet*, **ii**, 749.

Malmros, H. and Wigand, G. (1960). *Z. Ernahrungswiss.* **1**, 20.

Middleton, C. C., Clarkson, T. B., Lofland, H. B. and Prichard, R. W. (1967). *Arch. Pathol.* **83**, 145.

Morin, R. J., Bernick, S. and Alfin-Slater, R. B. (1964). *J. Atheroscler. Res.* **4**, 387.

Olson, R. E. (1958). *Perspec. Biol. Med.* **2**, 84.

O'Neal, R. M., Still, W. J. S. and Hartroft, W. S. (1961). *J. Pathol. Bacteriol.* **82**, 183.

Page, I. H. and Brown, H. B. (1952). *Circulation*, **6**, 681.

Patek, P. R., Bernick, S., Ershoff, B. H. and Wells, A. (1963). *Amer. J. Pathol.* **42**, 137.

Portman, O. W. and Andrus, S. B. (1965). *J. Nutr.* **87**, 429.

Rinehart, J. F. and Greenberg, L. D. (1949). *Amer. J. Pathol.* **25**, 481.

Roberts, J. C. and Straus, R. (1965). "Comparative Atherosclerosis". Hoeber Medical Division, Harper and Row, New York.

Rowsell, H. C., Downie, H. G. and Mustard, J. F. (1958). *Can. Med. Ass. J.* **79**, 647.

Rowsell, H. C., Downie, H. G. and Mustard, J. F. (1960). *Can. Med. Ass. J.* **83**, 1175.

Saltykow, S. (1908). *Zentr. Allg. Pathol. Pathol. Anat.* **19**, 321.

Scebat, L., Renais, J. and Lenegre, J. (1961). *Rev. Atherosclerose*, **3**, no. 2, 14.

Shull, K. H. and Mann, G. V. (1957). *Amer. J. Physiol.* **188**, 81.

Skold, B. H. and Getty, R. (1961). *J. Amer. Vet. Med. Ass.* **139**, 655.

Stamler, J., Pick, R. and Katz, L. N. (1959). *Circ. Res.* **7**, 398.

Steiner, A. and Kendall, F. E. (1946). *Arch. Pathol.* **42**, 433.

Steiner, A., Kendall, F. E. and Bevans, M. (1949). *Amer. Heart J.* **38**, 34.

Still, W. J. S. and O'Neal, R. M. (1962). *Amer. J. Pathol.* **40**, 21.

Strong, J. P. and McGill, H. C. (1967). *Amer. J. Pathol.* **50**, 669.

Taylor, C. B., Cox, G. E., Manalo-Estrella, P. and Southworth, J. (1962). *Arch. Pathol.* **74**, 16.

Taylor, C. B., Manalo-Estrella, P. and Cox, G. E. (1963). *Arch. Pathol.* **76**, 239.

Thomas, W. A., Scott, R. F., Lee, K. T., Daoud, A. S. and Jones, R. M. (1965). *In* "Comparative Atherosclerosis" (Eds J. C. Roberts and R. Straus), p. 92. Hoeber Medical Division, Harper and Row, New York.

Vles, R. D., Buller, J., Gottenbos, J. J. and Thomasson, H. J. (1964). *J. Atheroscler. Res.* **4**, 170.

Wacker, I. and Hueck, W. (1913). *Muench. Med. Wochenschr.* **60**, 2097.

Wesselkin, N. W. (1913). *Arch. Pathol. Anat. Physiol.* **212**, 225.

Wissler, R. W., Frazier, L. E., Hughes, R. H. and Rasmussen, R. A. (1962). *Arch. Pathol.* **74**, 312.

Hyperlipidaemia and the Pathogenesis of Atherosclerosis[1]

K. W. WALTON, MD, PhD, MRCS, FRCPath

Department of Experimental Pathology, University of Birmingham, England

1 Involvement of low-density and very low-density lipoproteins in atherogenesis

The atherosclerotic plaque at various stages of its development, and wherever it occurs in the arterial tree, is characterized by lipid deposition. Earlier suggestions that the lipid is derived from breakdown ("fatty metamorphosis") of intrinsic components of the arterial wall (Thoma, 1883), or originates from blood clots or cellular components of the blood deposited on the surface and later incorporated into the wall (Rokitansky, 1952) are no longer widely entertained (for reviews, see Walton, 1969a; 1973a). Instead, current research appears broadly to validate the view put forward by Virchow (1862) that the lipid originates from the plasma by a process of "imbibition" or "insudation".

The insudative theory was given impetus when it was shown by Anitschkow (1913) that the addition of cholesterol to the diet of rabbits gives rise to hypercholesterolaemia accompanied by the development of lesions resembling those seen in the human, which are rich in cholesterol. As a result, from that time on and until today a great deal of attention has been focused on this sterol and its distribution in the blood and tissues. However, neither cholesterol itself nor the other serum lipids (triglycerides and phospholipids) are water-soluble. They therefore cannot circulate in the free state but occur in the plasma bound to proteins in various forms (chylomicra, low-, very low-, and high-density lipoproteins).

[1] Based on communication given at Symposium "Perspectives in Ischaemic Heart Disease", Society for Drug Research, London, 26–27 September 1973.

The available evidence suggests that, among these various kinds of plasma lipid-carrying proteins, it is the low-density (LDL) and very low-density (VLDL) lipoproteins rather than chylomicra or high-density (HDL) lipoproteins which are of greatest importance in atherogenesis. The evidence is both indirect (correlative) and direct. For example:

a. Indirect evidence

i. Differences in total low-density (LDL + VLDL) levels with age and sex parallel differences in serum cholesterol levels and differences in the incidence of atherosclerosis with age and sex in a given community (Walton and Scott, 1964—and see Fig. 1). From this Figure it can be seen, firstly, that there is a divergence in serum cholesterol levels between the sexes which is broadly parallel to the similar divergence in total low-density lipoprotein levels, but unrelated to HDL

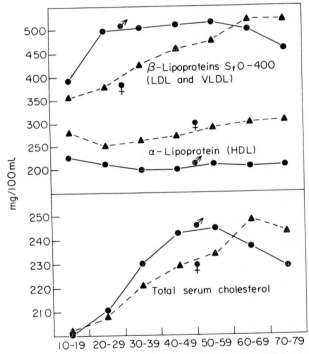

FIG. 1. Variation with age and sex of mean serum concentrations of total low- and very low-density lipoproteins and of high-density lipoprotein as compared with mean total serum cholesterol. Note similar shapes of curves for LDL and VLDL and for serum total cholesterol. (From Walton, 1973a.) (Reproduced with permission.)

levels (which show little change with age), suggesting that LDL and VLDL are the principal vehicles for cholesterol. The significance of this is that previous epidemiological data in which serum cholesterol alone has been measured can be interpreted, without significant error, to imply similar changes in LDL + VLDL levels. In disease, serum cholesterol elevations are likewise always reflected in increases in LDL and/or VLDL and *not* in high-density lipoproteins. Secondly, the time-scale over which the divergence in serum cholesterol or LDL levels occurs corresponds with the period of reproductive activity during which the incidence of atherosclerosis in women is known to be lower than in men.

ii. Geographical differences in the incidence of atherosclerosis between communities in different locations in the world are paralleled by differences in the mean serum LDL and VLDL (or cholesterol) levels between the same communities (Morris and Gardner, 1969). It can be seen from Table 1, for instance, that there is a broad relation between

TABLE 1

Relation between percentage involvement of intimal surface of coronary artery involved by raised atherosclerotic lesions (RL) and ranking order of local mean serum cholesterol or of proportion of dietary calories from fat for different locations[a]

Location (race, group)	RL	Ranking by serum cholesterol	% calories from fat
New Orleans—white	18·3	1	2
Oslo	17·8	2	1
New Orleans—negro	14·5	3	4
Manila	12·8	6	6
Puerto Rico	9·4	4	3
Cali	9·1	8	11
Lima	8·5	10	5
San Jose	8·4	11	12
Santiago	8·2	5	10
Bogota	6·7	9	8
Guatemala	6·5	12	9
Durban—Bantu	6·2	7	7

[a] From Morris and Gardner (1969).

the mean percentage of intimal surface involved of a given reference vessel (coronary artery) and the rank order for serum cholesterol levels for a given population. It can also be inferred from this Table that environmental rather than ethnic factors are involved and that probably an environmental factor of significance is the average intake of calories as fat in the diet by a given population.

iii. Otherwise pathologically disparate conditions secondarily associated with high serum LDL and/or VLDL levels (hypothyroidism, the nephrotic syndrome, obstructive biliary disease, chronic alcoholism) nevertheless share in common a tendency to a high incidence of atherosclerotic disease and its complications (for references, see Walton, 1973a). A similar tendency is also seen in certain primary (familial) hyperlipidaemias. Studies of the turnover and distribution of LDL in both primary and secondary hyperlipidaemias (Walton, 1969b) have established that although the *mechanisms* underlying the elevation of the hyperlipidaemia may differ (see Table 2), the common factor is an

TABLE 2

Turnover and distribution of LDL in health and hyperlipidaemia as derived from studies with radioactively labelled LDL

Category		Sex	Mean serum LDL (mg/100 ml)	Pool size IV^a (mg kg^{-1})	Pool size EV^b (mg kg^{-1})	Catabolic rate (mg kg^{-1} day^{-1})	$T_B{}^c$ (days)
Healthy		M	558	174	87	59	3·5
		F	513	280	140	98	2·4
Secondary hyper-	Hypothyroid	F	1475	500	250	63	6·0
lipidaemia	Nephrotic	M	1192	473	336	146	3·6
Primary	Type IIA	M	920	790	395	182	2·9
(familial)	Type III	M	1502	839	429	223	3·1
hyper- lipidaemia	Type IV	M	1020	739	369	147	3·3

[a] IV, intravascular pool.   [b] EV, extravascular pool.   [c] T_B, biological half-life.

increase in total body pool of LDL. It seems possible that, in particular, the increase of extravascular pool is given expression as deposition of LDL in arterial walls and in other sites in the body (*e.g.* xanthomata—see Scott and Winterbourn, 1967).

In the case of primary hyperlipidaemias, it is noteworthy that Types II-V (according to the classification of Fredrickson *et al.*, 1967), all of which are characterized by raised levels of LDL and/or VLDL, show an increased incidence of cardiovascular disease (CVD), whereas Type I, which is characterized by gross chylomicronaemia but *low* levels of LDL and VLDL, does not show any increased incidence of CVD. This suggests that chylomicra are not atherogenic. Presumably this is either because they are too large in particle size to enter the arterial wall, or if they do enter, because they are disposed of too rapidly to evoke a response in the arterial connective tissue.

b.   Direct evidence

iv. In certain instances in which autologous LDL, radioactively labelled in its protein moiety, has been administered *in vivo* and subsequent autopsy examination has been possible, it has been shown (Walton *et al.*, 1963—see Table 3; Scott and Hurley, 1970) that

TABLE 3

Distribution of radioactivity in tissues[a]

Tissue	Radioactivity (counts s^{-1} g^{-1} tissue)
Brachial nerve plexus	0·34
Myocardium	0·36
Adipose tissue	1·04
Brachial artery	1·08
Liver tissue	1·226
(two specimens counted)	1·232
Spleen	1·231
Coronary artery	1·74
Aorta	2·62
(two portions counted)	2·62
Aortic intima (from area of atheromatous infiltration)	3·28
Serum	30·60 counts s^{-1} ml^{-1}

[a] At autopsy on patient dying of ischaemic heart disease during course (9th day) of turnover study with autologous radio-iodinated LDL—see Walton *et al.* (1963).

atherosclerotic vessels accumulate radioactivity at a higher level per gram of tissue than other organs, suggesting that circulating LDL enters the vessel wall by an insudative process.

v. Confirmation of the entry of LDL and VLDL into atherosclerotic lesions (but absence of HDL in the same lesions) has also been obtained at a histological level (Figs 2–4) using immunofluorescence (Walton and Williamson, 1968; Walton, 1974a). In this work the distribution of extracellular lipid in lesions (as delineated by conventional fat stains) was found to correspond exactly with the distribution

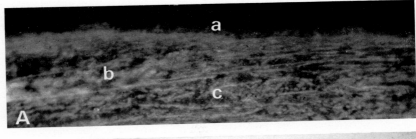

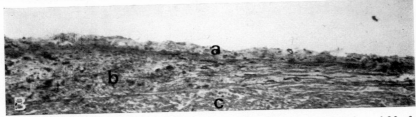

FIG. 2. (A) Frozen section through "fatty streak" from aorta of girl aged 23 after treatment with fluorescein-labelled anti-LDL and examination in ultraviolet light. In the original, specific bright green fluorescence was visible in endothelial cells (a) and intimal layer (b), contrasting with blue autofluorescence in muscular layer (c). (B) Same field of same section stained for lipid. Note correspondence between distribution of lipid (dark grey or black in picture, bright red in original) with areas giving fluorescence (a and b) in (A). Oil red O, haematoxylin, light green. Magnification × 375.

of LDL or VLDL as shown by the immunological technique. The significance of this observation is that fat stains react only with the lipid portion of lipoproteins and not with the protein. Conversely, the antibody is directed mainly or exclusively against the protein portion. Precise topographic correspondence between the two techniques thus makes it reasonable to infer that the intact lipoprotein molecule must be present in the lesion.

Using antisera specific for other individual plasma proteins the only other protein found significantly to be related to atherosclerotic lesions was fibrinogen (Walton and Williamson, 1968).

vi. In relation to experimental models, it has been shown that whether rabbits are maintained on diets supplemented with cholesterol, or with beef-fat without added cholesterol, the animals develop increased levels of LDL and/or VLDL. The arterial lesions in these animals, as in the human, contain lipid which can be shown by immunofluorescence to be associated with these lipoproteins (Walton, 1973b; 1974b). This suggests that, in relation to their response to hyperlipoproteinaemia, such animals serve as a valid model for an insudative process in the

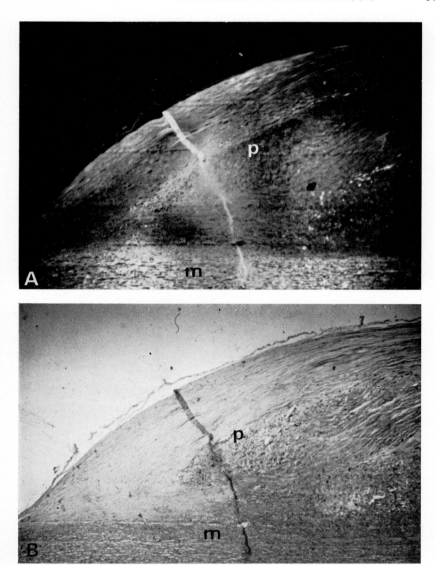

FIG. 3. (A) Frozen section through large fibro-fatty aortic plaque, from man aged 47, after treatment with fluorescein-labelled anti-LDL. In the original, bright green specific fluorescence (greyish-white in picture) seen in plaque (p) contrasting with blue autofluorescence of media (m). *Note* the oblique line crossing the plaque is a fold in the section. (B) Same field of same section stained for lipid. *Note* correspondence between lipid (grey in picture, bright red in original) on surface of collagen in plaque in this picture and distribution of specific fluorescence in (A) in plaque. Oil red O, haematoxylin, light green. Magnification × 125.

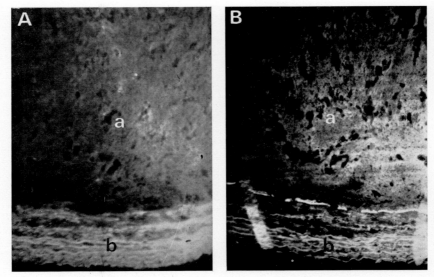

FIG. 4. (A) Frozen section of portion of plaque in mouth of renal artery, from man of 55, after treatment with fluorescein-labelled anti-HDL. In the original, blue autofluorescence (negative reaction) seen in both plaque (a) and in media (b). (B) Consecutive frozen section from same material after treatment with fluorescein-labelled anti-LDL. In the original, bright green specific fluorescence seen in plaque (a) contrasting with blue autofluorescence in media (b). Magnification × 375.

human although in other respects (e.g. grossly disordered cholesterol metabolism) they are less satisfactory.

2 Mechanism of lipid retention in atherosclerotic lesions

The selective retention of plasma lipids in the arterial intima has been suggested to be due to various alternative mechanisms. These include (for references, see Walton, 1973a):

    a. changes in the tunica media following (i) blockage of fenestrations in the internal elastic lamina, (ii) scarring of the muscularis media, (iii) enzymic medial defects due to anoxia; or

    b. failure of lipids (lipoproteins) to permeate through the intima because of a "molecular sieving" effect of the intimal connective tissue gel; or

    c. interaction of LDL and VLDL with the sulphated glycosaminoglycans (S-GAGs) of the intimal connective tissue.

In relation to these suggested mechanisms, consideration of the evidence outlined above leads one to submit, firstly, that sub-endothelial lipid accumulation cannot be due to a mechanical barrier effect since this would be expected to cause accumulation of *all* the protein components of plasma (including HDL) whereas a selective retention is found; and also because LDL is demonstrable in very early lesions ("fatty streaks" and "spots") *before* changes in the elastic lamina or media are demonstrable (Walton, 1973c). For similar reasons, a "molecular sieving" retention seems unlikely to apply.

On the other hand these studies suggest that it is something in the *nature of the vehicle* for lipids (i.e. some aspect of the physicochemical characteristics of LDL and VLDL) rather than the nature of the lipids themselves that determines initial localization. It would seem likely that fibrinogen, the only other plasma protein significantly related to lesion formation, would share such characteristics.

In this connection it has been shown that the only plasma proteins which selectively form insoluble complexes *in vitro* with the S-GAGs of the arterial connective tissues are LDL, VLDL and fibrinogen (Amenta and Waters, 1960; Gerö *et al.*, 1960). Moreover, studies using histochemical methods (Curran and Crane, 1962) or techniques employing radiosulphate uptake (Gerö *et al.*, 1967) have shown a correlation between the distribution of S-GAGs and that of lipid (LDL) in atherosclerotic lesions.

It is now well established that plasma proteins *normally* permeate through the walls of the aorta and of arteries (Mancini *et al.*, 1962; Duncan *et al.*, 1962; Scott and Hurley, 1970) draining into lymphatics in the outer coat. Because of the observations outlined above, it has been proposed that during the passage of plasma through the connective tissue gel, LDL and VLDL and fibrinogen are selectively retained in the gel by interaction with the S-GaGs present in the gel and that calcium ions also play a part in this process (for further discussion, see Walton and Williamson, 1968; Walton, 1969a; 1973d).

3   Factors affecting LDL deposition in arteries

In terms of the concept outlined above, it is clear that (*a*) increasing inflow of plasma into the arterial wall (increased permeability, hypertension), or (*b*) conditions associated with altered composition of the plasma (hyperlipoproteinaemia), or (*c*) conditions restricting outflow (obstruction to the lymphatic drainage of the wall), would all contribute to the accumulation of LDL, VLDL and/or fibrinogen in the gel. From this viewpoint, the manner in which certain known clinical "risk factors" might operate and mutually reinforce one another in influencing the occurrence of arterial disease is indicated in Table 4.

TABLE 4

Possible mechanism whereby known clinical "risk factors" operate

Risk factors	Possible mechanism
1. Age, smoking (hypoxia) extrinsic or intrinsic vaso-active agents	Moderate hyperlipoproteinaemia with age in presence of increased permeability (increased inflow into arterial wall)
2. Hypertension	Increased "ultra-filtration" of plasma (increased inflow ± hyperlipoproteinaemia)
3. Sex, diet, ?genetic predisposition to high intestinal fat absorption	Moderate hyperlipoproteinaemia (increased input of LDL even with unchanged volume of inflow)
4. Hyperlipidaemia of familial origin or secondary to diabetes, nephrosis, etc.	Gross hyperlipoproteinaemia (marked increase of input of LDL even with unchanged volume of inflow)
5. Previous or coexistent granulomatous arterial disease	Inflammation of wall increasing vascular permeability; distortion of lymphatic drainage reducing arterial outflow

For example, in relation to increased permeability, in old age (the eighth and ninth decades of life), in addition to discrete but discontinuous atherosclerotic plaques, the sub-endothelial tissues in apparently *unaffected* areas of the aorta, cerebral and coronary arteries show diffuse lipid (lipoprotein) infiltration (Fig. 5). This possibly reflects the increased permeability of membranes which is a generalized phenomenon in old age. But a similar change is sometimes seen precociously in heavy cigarette smokers (Fig. 6). It has been shown that an appreciable chronic carboxyhaemoglobinaemia is found in heavy smokers (Kjeldsen, 1970) and it seems possible that this form of hypoxia induces generalized alteration of vascular permeability to account for the findings alluded to above. The role of altered permeability in determining extravascular lipid deposits (xanthomata and the corneal arcus), which are broadly correlated with atherosclerosis, has been discussed elsewhere (Walton *et al.*, 1973; Walton, 1973c).

Hypertension, whether naturally occurring in man or experimentally induced in laboratory animals, is known to accelerate the development of atherosclerosis, especially in the presence of hyperlipidaemia (for references, see Walton, 1969a). The occurrence of lipid (LDL) deposition in

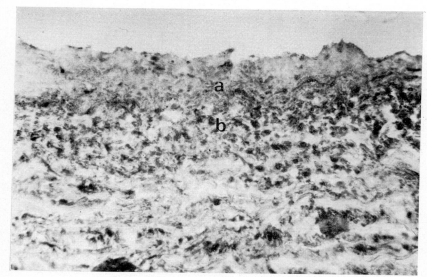

FIG. 5. Frozen section of portion of aorta *unaffected* by naked-eye evidence of atherosclerosis from woman aged 86. Lipid diffusely distributed as droplets (grey or black in picture, bright red in original) in superficial (a) and deeper portions (b) of thickened intima. Oil red O, haematoxylin and light green. Magnification × 375.

valves on the left side of the heart, which are at arterial pressure, and not in valves on the right side of the heart, which are at venous pressure, mirrors the occurrence of lipid deposition in arteries but not in veins and emphasizes the role of haemodynamic pressure in determining "ultrafiltration" of plasma and thereby the sites of LDL accumulation (Walton *et al.*, 1970; Walton, 1973c).

Lastly, preexistent or coincident arterial disease affecting the arterial wall (syphilitic arteritis, granulomatous arteritis) are known to be associated with increased atherosclerosis. External injury to arteries also causes localization of plaques to the overlying intima. It seems probable that these processes, which result in distortion or blockage of lymphatic drainage of the wall, would decrease outflow of plasma from the wall, thus allowing LDL and fibrinogen to be entrained in the connective tissue gel.

4   Summary

Hyperlipidaemia has long been known to be broadly correlated with the occurrence of atherosclerosis. Since lipids are water insoluble and are carried in the plasma as complex molecules, the lipoproteins, in practice, hyperlipidaemia is invariably an expression of hyperlipoproteinaemia.

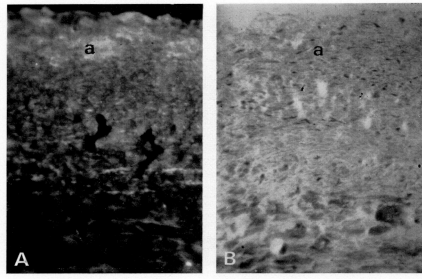

FIG. 6. (A) Frozen section of portion of coronary artery *unaffected* by naked-eye evidence of atherosclerosis from man of 37 who had habitually smoked 45 cigarettes per day. Section treated with fluorescein-labelled anti-LDL. In original, bright-green fluorescence (pale-grey in picture) seen in superficial portion (a) of thickened intima. (B) Consecutive section from same material, stained for lipid. Finely dispersed lipid droplets (grey in picture, bright red in original) seen in area corresponding to distribution of specific fluorescence in (A). Oil red O, haematoxylin, light green. Magnification × 375.

Current evidence is reviewed which suggests that, of the various lipoproteins present in plasma, it is the low- and very low-density lipoproteins which are implicated in atherogenesis and that these proteins enter the arterial wall by an insudative process, being selectively retained in the connective tissue gel by interaction with the sulphated glycosaminoglycans of the gel.

Other factors contributing to lipoprotein deposition in the arterial wall (increased permeability, hypertension and impaired drainage of the arterial wall) are also considered in relation to the way in which these mechanisms may underlie known clinical "risk factors" accepted as influencing the occurrence of arterial disease.

References

Amenta, J. S. and Waters, L. L. (1960). *Yale J. Biol. Med.* **33**, 112.
Anitschkow, N. (1913). *Beitr. Pathol. Anat.* **56**, 379.
Curran, R. C. and Crane, W. A. J. (1962). *J. Pathol. Bacteriol.* **84**, 405.

Duncan, L. E., Cornfield, J. and Buck, K. (1962). *J. Clin. Invest.* **41**, 1537.
Gerö, S., Gergely, J., Dévényi, T., Jakab, L., Székely, J. and Virág, S. (1960). *Nature (London)*, **187**, 152.
Gerö, S., Virág, S., Bihari-Varga, M., Székely, J. and Feher, J. (1967). *In* "Progress in Biochemical Pharmacology" (Eds D. Kritchevsky, R. Paoletti and D. Steinberg), vol. 2, p. 290. Karger, Basel.
Kjeldsen, K. (1970). *In* "Atherosclerosis: Proceedings of the Second International Symposium" (Ed. R. J. Jones), p. 378. Springer-Verlag, Berlin.
Mancini, R. E., Vilar, O., Dellacha, J. M., Davidson, O. W., Gomez, C. J. and Alvarez, B., (1962). *J. Histochem. Cytochem.* **10**, 194.
Morris, J. N. and Gardner, M. J. (1969). *Amer. J. Med.* **46**, 674.
Rokitansky, C. von (1952). *In* "A Manual of Pathological Anatomy" (Translated by G. E. Day), vol. 4, p. 261. Sydenham Society, London.
Scott, P. J. and Hurley, P. J. (1970). *Atherosclerosis*, **11**, 77.
Scott, P. J. and Winterbourn, C. C. (1967). *J. Atheroscler. Res.* **7**, 207.
Thoma, R. (1883). *Virchows Arch. Pathol. Anat. Physiol.* **93**, 443.
Virchow, R. (1862). *In* "Gesammelte Abhandlungen zur wissenschaftlichen Medizin". Max Hirsch, Berlin.
Walton, K. W. (1969a). *In* "The Biological Basis of Medicine" (Eds E. Bittar and N. Bittar), vol. 6, p. 193. Academic Press, London and New York.
Walton, K. W. (1969b). *In* "Physiology and Pathophysiology of Plasma Proteins" (Eds G. Birke, R. Norburg and L. O. Plantin), p. 145. Pergamon Press, Oxford.
Walton, K. W. (1973a). *In* "Textbook of Geriatric Medicine and Gerontology" (Ed. J. C. Brocklehurst), p. 77. Churchill-Livingstone, London.
Walton, K. W. (1973b). *In* "Connective Tissue and Ageing" (Ed. H. G. Vogel), p. 42. Excerpta Medica, Amsterdam.
Walton, K. W. (1973c). *In* "Connective Tissue and Ageing" (Ed. H. G. Vogel), p. 34. Excerpta Medica, Amsterdam.
Walton, K. W. (1973d). *In* "Connective Tissue and Ageing" (Ed. H. G. Vogel), p. 21. Excerpta Medica, Amsterdam.
Walton, K. W. (1973e). *Nutr. Metabol.* **15**, 37.
Walton, K. W. (1974a). *In* "Proceedings of IIIrd International Symposium on Atherosclerosis". Springer-Verlag, Berlin. (In press.)
Walton, K. W. (1974b). *In* "Proceedings of IIIrd International Symposium on Atherosclerosis". Springer-Verlag, Berlin. (In press.)
Walton, K. W. and Scott, P. J. (1964). *J. Clin. Pathol.* **17**, 627.
Walton, K. W. and Williamson, N. (1968). *J. Atheroscler. Res.* **8**, 599.
Walton, K. W., Scott, P. J., Verrier-Jones, J., Fletcher, R. F. and Whitehead, T. P. (1963). *J. Atheroscler. Res.* **3**, 396.
Walton, K. W., Williamson, N. and Johnson, A. G. (1970). *J. Pathol.* **101**, 205.
Walton, K. W., Thomas, C. and Dunkerley, D. J. (1973). *J. Pathol.* **109**, 271.

Electrophysiological Basis for a Rational Approach to Antidysrhythmic Drug Therapy

E. M. VAUGHAN WILLIAMS, DM, DSc

Department of Pharmacology, University of Oxford, England

1 Introduction

In the highly developed countries mortality from cardiovascular disease is extremely high. Although there are regional differences (for example, in Japan cerebral vascular disease predominates, whereas in Europe and the USA the heart is the primary target) a satisfactory explanation for such variations is not available. What is certain is that vascular deterioration starts early in life and is progressive. Postmortem examinations performed on battle casualties, accident victims and people meeting other kinds of violent death, have revealed that atheromatous plaques begin to form in the coronaries of quite young persons, in their twenties and thirties. By the age of 50 half the population, even without any symptoms of cardiac disease, have at least one coronary artery occluded by 50 per cent or more, and less than one fifth have entirely unoccluded arteries at this age (Rissanen, 1970). Until about ten years ago fibrillation and severe dysrhythmias were not especially associated with coronary thrombosis, but since the introduction of continuous ECG recording 24 hours a day in intensive care units it has become evident that 95 per cent of patients with cardiac infarction exhibit some episode of dysrhythmia within the first 48 hours (Julian *et al.*, 1964). One of the most puzzling features of postmortem examinations of cardiac infarctions was that so many people, especially the younger ones, had died in spite of the fact that the mass of ventricular tissue deprived of its blood supply was often quite small. The implication was that these patients had succumbed to ventricular fibrillation, and that the immediate availability of a really safe and effective antidysrhythmic drug could have prolonged a number of lives.

Thus the urgent need for further research into the production of new antidysrhythmic compounds can hardly be in doubt. Unfortunately, when one looks for a rational basis upon which a systematic investigation might be founded, the situation is hopelessly confused. There is not even agreement about the classification of the drugs we already have. Vaughan Williams (1970b) categorized known antidysrhythmic agents according to their individual electrophysiological and pharmacological actions, emphasizing that some compounds had more than one class of action. In the following year Bassett and Hoffman (1971) produced a quite different classification, but did not mention the earlier one, an omission unhelpful to a clinician seeking enlightenment.

Another difficulty impeding the development of new drugs is the lack of a reliable animal model for the study of dysrhythmias. Abnormalities of cardiac rhythm can be produced experimentally by a variety of methods— aconitine, chloroform and adrenaline, acetylcholine and electrical stimulation, overdosage with digitalis, coronary ligation etc.—but such procedures are unreliable and offer no guarantee that results obtained with them are relevant to clinical situations in man. For this reason it was decided about fifteen years ago to approach the problem from the opposite end, as it were, and to study in detail the electrophysiological and other effects of drugs which were *known* to be antidysrhythmic in man, in the hope of finding some accurately measurable common actions. The objective of a search for hard facts about the properties of such agents was twofold. First a screen for new compounds could be designed, because if a new compound also possessed similar properties it would be likely to be antidysrhythmic. Secondly, a detailed study of the mode of action of drugs capable of controlling dysrhythmias might throw some light on the cellular basis of the dysrhythmias themselves.

Thus in this paper no attempt will be made to discuss in detail the relative clinical effectiveness of available antidysrhythmic drugs in different types of dysrhythmias. It is proposed, instead, to start from the beginning and to discuss fundamental aspects of excitability in cardiac muscle; to describe the actual electrophysiological and pharmacological properties of the main classes of antidysrhythmic drugs; to indicate how their actions could be effective in terms of current theories concerning the origin of dysrhythmias, and finally to suggest how the clinical approach to therapy could be set upon a more rational basis in the light of this evidence.

2 Electrophysiology of cardiac muscle

Much of our knowledge of the biophysical basis of excitation and contraction has come from studies of the behaviour of the squid giant axon and frog sartorius muscle. It is probable that the fundamental processes are similar in cardiac muscle, but there are important differences which require emphasis. Although detailed accounts are available elsewhere, it may be helpful to recapitulate briefly the main points before discussing the mode of action of antidysrhythmic drugs.

It has been known for a couple of generations that the interior of nerves and muscles is negatively charged at rest, the electromotive force (EMF) being provided by the relatively high intracellular concentration of potassium ions (E_K). Hodgkin and his colleagues, however, found that during the action potential the inside of nerves actually became positive relative to the outside (Hodgkin, 1958). Thus there had to be two batteries, not one. They suggested that the second EMF was provided by the concentration difference of sodium ions, high outside, low inside. At rest this sodium battery (E_{Na}) remained switched off, as it were, but activation was associated with a large increase in sodium permeability, so that a positive charge of sodium ions entered the cell. This action was very brief, lasting less than a millisecond, after which the sodium permeability was inactivated, and the Na-battery switched off again. The importance of this inactivation of sodium permeability was that the membrane would remain absolutely refractory to the passage of further sodium currents until the processes just described had been reversed by repolarization. This may be illustrated by reference to an actual cardiac action potential (Figs 1a and 1b).

The refractory period in cardiac muscle is extremely long, because *re*polarization is about 100 times slower than *de*polarization. In order to measure the rate of *de*polarization, therefore, it is necessary to look at the intracellularly recorded potentials at a faster sweep speed. The process of activation or depolarization has three phases. At rest (inside potential negative) sodium permeability is low, as though a gate in the membrane (labelled m) were closed. When current from a neighbouring active

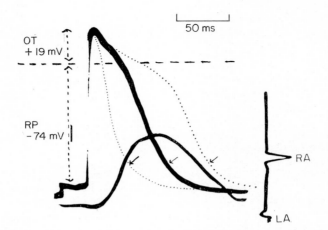

Fig. 1a. Cardiac action potential. —————— Zero potential with electrode outside fibre. *Centre trace* electrode inside single cardiac cell showing resting potential (RP) − 74 mV. The stimulus in a distant fibre on the left atrium appears as an artifact. When the active region reaches the cell in which the electrode is situated, the inside becomes positive (overshoot, Ot) by +19 mV and slowly repolarizes. The arrows indicate the point of repolarization at which a second response would be possible, and the dotted lines indicate that any drug or condition which accelerated or delayed repolarization would shorten or lengthen the absolute refractory period. *Vertical trace, right:* externally recorded action potentials from left (LA) and right (RA) atria from which conduction velocity may be calculated. *Bottom trace:* contraction.

region depolarizes a fibre (phase 1), something occurs in the membrane so that permeability to sodium increases (the m-gate opens) and in phase 2 the fibre itself becomes actively depolarized, and begins passively to depolarize the next fibre so that the action potential propagates. Finally (phase 3) the sodium permeability is inactivated, as though another gate (labelled h), in series with the first, became closed. The membrane will thus remain absolutely refractory to sodium current until repolarization has made it possible for the h-gate to reopen. It is at once apparent that any drug or condition which shortened the duration of the cardiac action potential would automatically shorten the refractory period, and so increase the probability of fibrillation. This is, in fact, the effect of acetylcholine, of hypoxia and of halogen anaesthetics, all known to be liable to precipitate dysrhythmias. Conversely, if repolarization were delayed, the refractory period would be prolonged.

So much for the introductory electrophysiology. We may now turn to the actual effects of the drugs themselves.

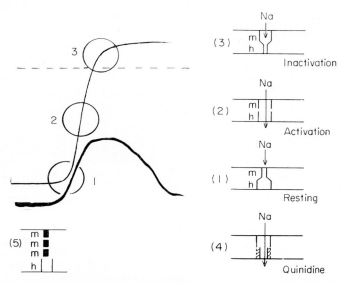

FIG. 1b. Cardiac action potential—intracellular record at a faster sweep. (1) Current flowing into approaching active region begins to repolarize fibre; *right*—at the resting potential the h gate is open, the m gate is closed. (2) Depolarization opens the m gate; Na current into the fibre is maximal. (3) Depolarization has closed the h gate, and Na current is inactivated. (4) Diagram to show that the action of quinidine may be to prevent the h gate reopening fully after repolarization, so that in stage 2 of a depolarization, maximum Na current is not reached. (5) Diagram showing that if three m gates are in series with one h gate, the instantaneous sodium conductance G_{Na}, expressed as a fraction of maximum conductance $\overline{G}_{Na}$, is given by $G_{Na} = \overline{G}_{Na}m^3h$: m and h have values between 0 and 1, and are functions of transmembrane voltage and time.

3 Pharmacology of antidysrhythmic drugs

3. CLASS I ACTION

There are certainly three and possibly four classes of antidysrhythmic action. Several drugs have more than one mode of action, and some confusion might have been avoided if a quantitative estimate had been available of the relative concentrations required to produce the respective effects.

Quinidine is the prototype of antidysrhythmic drugs, and its electrophysiological effects on heart muscle may be considered the first class of antidysrhythmic action.

Quinidine causes no change in the resting potential, and thus presumably does not interfere with the metabolic processes responsible for ion-pumping across the membrane, so that the potassium battery

Quinidine (+ -isomer)

remains fully charged (Vaughan Williams, 1958a). The intracellular concentration of potassium is not lowered by quinidine, nor is the intracellular sodium concentration raised (Goodford and Vaughan Williams, 1962). Nevertheless the maximum rate of depolarization (MRD) was greatly reduced in the presence of quinidine, in spite of the fact that the driving force for depolarization (the voltage of the sodium battery, E_{Na}) was unaffected. It must be assumed, therefore, that quinidine had some direct effect on the membrane, restricting the entry of depolarization current, as though it were obstructing the full opening of one of the "gates" (Fig. 1b).

One might ask why should a drug which reduces the rate of entry of depolarization current be antifibrillatory? It has been known for a long time that owing to the process of accommodation in excitable tissues, very slowly rising currents fail to excite. Thus, a minimum rate of depolarization must be achieved in order for an action potential to be propagated. It has already been mentioned that repolarization has to occur before the h-gate can re-open and permit the entry of sodium ions for a second action potential. The effective refractory may be defined as the point at which the h-gate has opened sufficiently for the rate of rise of a second spike to be fast enough for propagation along the whole muscle to occur. The absolute refractory period is a little shorter than this, because a stimulus may produce a local response, even though the rate of rise is not fast enough for propagation (Fig. 2: diagram, left). In the presence of quinidine and other class I drugs the entry of depolarizing current is restricted, and repolarization has, therefore, to proceed much further before the gates are open wide enough for the minimum rate of rise for propagation to be reached. Thus the effective refractory period is prolonged by quinidine even though the duration of the action potential itself is not. It was shown (Vaughan Williams, 1961) that quinidine reduced the rate of rise of the action potential much more at high than at low frequencies of stimulation. It is thus antifibrillatory because it cuts out the propagation of the abnormal high frequency impulses, but not of the normal lower frequency sinus rhythm.

Quinidine, and other similarly acting compounds are also local anaesthetics on nerve but it must be emphasized that the concentration

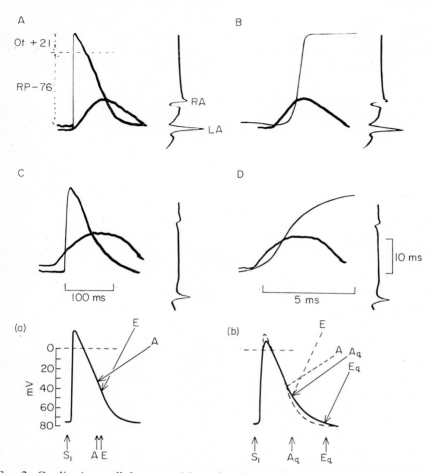

FIG. 2. Cardiac intracellular potentials at slow (A and C) and fast (B and D) sweep speeds. Contractions (*lower traces*) and externally recorded action potentials (*vertical traces*) are also shown. Effect of quinidine, 9 mg l^{-1}: (C) no change in resting potential, and the tail of repolarization is slightly prolonged. The contraction is dispersed in time, but not reduced and the conduction velocity is greatly slowed; (D) MRD is much slower. (a) Tracing of control action potential in response to a stimulus, S_1. A second stimulus at A causes a local response, but the rate of rise is not fast enough for propagation (the arrow is drawn tangentially to MRD at this point). When repolarization has proceeded to point E, the rate of rise is sufficiently fast for propagation. The interval S_1 to E is the effective refractory period. (b) Tracing of action potential in presence of quinidine (superimposed on control in dashed line). Although the duration of repolarization itself is little affected, direct interference with the mechanism of depolarization makes it necessary for repolarization to proceed to point E_q before MRD is fast enough for propagation, and the effective refractory period is prolonged greatly.

of the antidysrhythmic drugs required to depress excitability in the heart is much lower than that required for the local anaesthesia of nerve. Therein lies their value. Quinidine, and other "class I" drugs with local anaesthetic action, such as procaine, procainamide and lignocaine, also depress cardiac contractions, but usually higher concentrations are required to depress contractions than to reduce the maximum rate of depolarization.

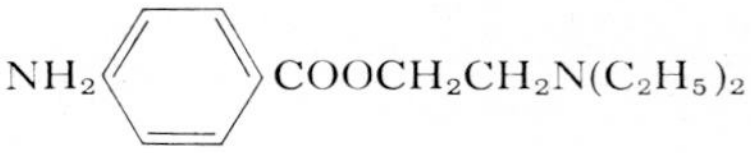

$$NH_2 \langle\bigcirc\rangle COOCH_2CH_2N(C_2H_5)_2$$

Procaine

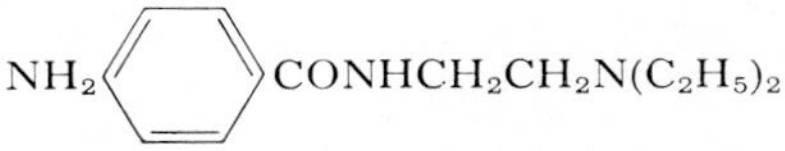

$$NH_2 \langle\bigcirc\rangle CONHCH_2CH_2N(C_2H_5)_2$$

Procainamide

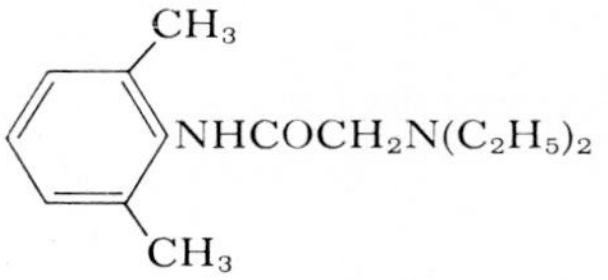

Lignocaine

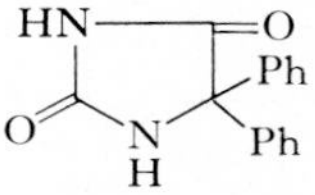

Diphenylhydantoin

The question must now be considered how lignocaine and diphenyl-hydantoin exert their antidysrhythmic action. Lignocaine is a well-known local anaesthetic, and one might naturally have supposed that it would act in the same way as procaine or procainamide and other drugs with local anaesthetic properties. It has been suggested, however, in particular by Davis and Temte in 1969, and Bigger and Mandel in 1970, that the antidysrhythmic actions of lignocaine and diphenylhydantoin are fundamentally different. Although these authors agreed that both drugs reduced the maximum rate of depolarization (MRD) of cardiac muscle, they claimed that higher concentrations were required to produce the effect than would occur in the blood of treated patients. We noted that the evidence on which this contention was based was obtained from tissues bathed with solutions very low in potassium. We have reinvestigated the electrophysiological effects of lignocaine and diphenylhydantoin both in low and in normal potassium solutions, and so far as the experimental observations are concerned, we have fully confirmed the findings of Bigger and his colleagues. At abnormally low potassium concentrations, higher concentrations of the drugs are needed to depress MRD. At a normal potassium concentration, however, both lignocaine and diphenylhydantoin depress MRD at concentrations well within the range found clinically (Fig. 3).

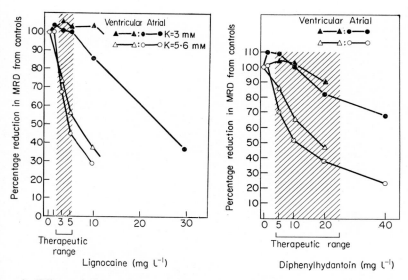

FIG. 3. Effect of lignocaine and diphenylhydantoin on the maximum rate of depolarization (MRD) of cardiac muscle in normal and low external potassium ion concentration. The control MRD is faster in low K than in normal K. Hatched areas indicate the range of concentrations of the drugs actually observed in the serum of successfully treated patients. Low potassium shifts the dose–response curves to the right, with the implication that a fall in serum K would prevent a patient responding to the drugs.

We have concluded, therefore, that lignocaine and diphenylhydantoin are probably antidysrhythmic because they depress MRD in common with other local anaesthetic type drugs (Singh and Vaughan Williams, 1971b). I would like to emphasize, however, that this is not to claim there are no differences between the actions of, say, quinidine and lignocaine in man or whole animals. On the contrary, there are several, especially in relation to their negative inotropic action, to their duration of action, to their atropine-like properties and to their effects on the central nervous system. So far as their direct effect on the cardiac membrane itself is concerned, however, there seems to be no reason to suppose that their mode of action is fundamentally different. We confirmed that low potassium caused a shift in the dose–response curve and this explains the clinical observations that lignocaine is ineffective in patients with low serum potassium (Pamintuan *et al.*, 1970).

3.2   CLASS II ACTION

It is well known that hyperactivity of the sympathetic system is liable to induce dysrhythmias and we may now turn to the second class of antidysrhythmic action, exhibited by drugs with antisympathetic effects, either by β-receptor blockade, or by interference with the release of sympathetic transmitters (bretylium, guanethidine). Such antisympathetic drugs would naturally be expected to be most effective in dysrhythmias associated with excessive sympathetic drive, but we found (Vaughan Williams and Sekiya, 1963) that β-receptor blocking drugs protected against ouabain-induced fibrillation also. This was in agreement with the finding of Méndez *et al.* (1961) that deprivation of sympathetic drive by sympathectomy and adrenalectomy prevented the occurrence of ventricular fibrillation after digitalis in dogs.

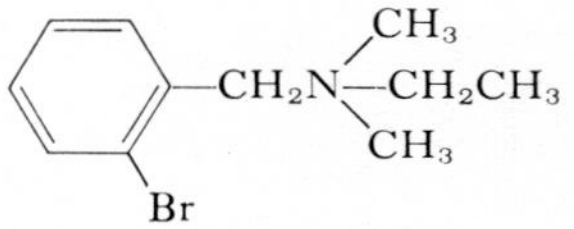

Bretylium

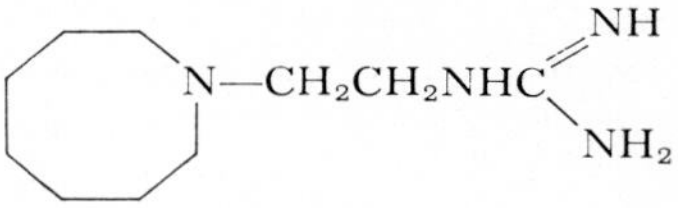

Guanethidine

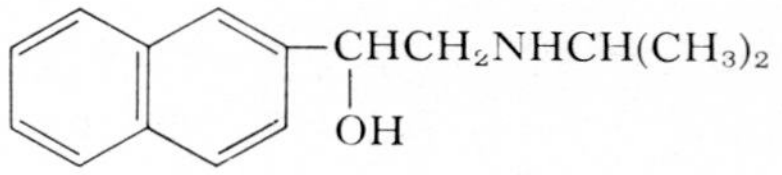

Pronethalol

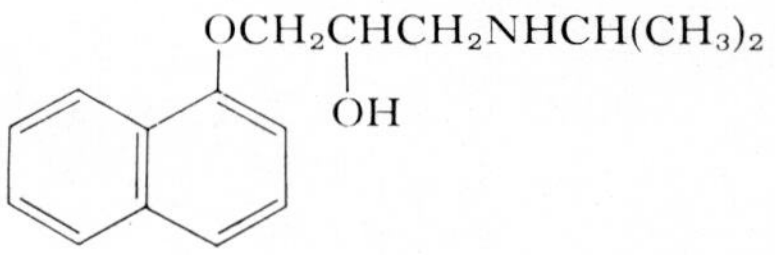

Propranolol

We soon discovered, however, that pronethalol and propranolol, and several other β-receptor blocking compounds, were powerful local anaesthetics, more potent than procaine. They also reduced the rate of rise of the action potential, as did the other antidysrhythmic drugs with local anaesthetic properties.

The question arose, therefore, whether β-receptor blockade had anything to do with the protection against digitalis, and some authors maintained that this action ("quinidine-like" or "class I") was sufficient to account for the prevention of digitalis-induced dysrhythmias. The laevo-isomer of propranolol, however, which has the same local anaesthetic potency as the dextro-isomer but is 100 times more active as a β-receptor blocker, was much more effective than the dextro-isomer in protecting against ouabain-induced ventricular fibrillation. There is much further recent evidence in favour of the original contention that antisympathetic drugs protect not only against dysrhythmias associated with excess sympathetic activity but also against those occurring after coronary ligation or digitalis intoxication (Dohadwalla, Freedberg and Vaughan Williams, 1969). Further support for this view is provided by the effect of bretylium. This drug blocks the release of noradrenaline from sympathetic nerve endings. It was also found to protect guinea pigs against ouabain-induced ventricular fibrillation (Papp and Vaughan Williams, 1969). When we looked at its electrophysiological properties, however, we found that it had no "class I" or direct membrane properties whatever (Fig. 4).

It is thus apparent that drugs with an antisympathetic action, whether produced by neurone blockade or by competition for transmitter at receptors, are antidysrhythmic in their own right, as it were. The removal of sympathetic background reduces the probability of dysrhythmia, whatever the precipitating factor may be.

3.3 CLASS III ACTION

In the hope of finding a lead for the development of new antidysrhythmic drugs, it was thought worthwhile to investigate the electrophysiological effects of conditions known to be associated with dysrhythmias. Hypoxia and halogen anaesthetics have already been mentioned. Now it is well established that hyperthyroidism causes atrial fibrillation, whereas in myxoedema, cardiac irregularities, apart from an occasional extra-systole associated with very low heart rates, are extremely rare. We have investigated the effects on cardiac intracellular potentials of hyper- and hypothyroidism. It was thought possible, for example, that in hypothyroidism, the rate of rise of the action potential might be reduced. It is

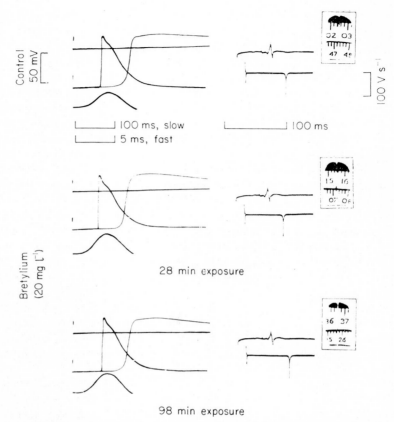

FIG. 4. The effect of bretylium on cardiac intracellular potentials. In each panel:
Left, horizontal trace, zero potential. *Middle traces,* intracellularly recorded potentials at slow and fast sweep speeds, superimposed. *Lower traces,* contractions.
Right, upper trace, stimulus artifact from electrode on left atrium, and externally
recorded action potential from external electrode on right atrium, for measurement
of conduction velocity. *Lower trace,* differentiated record (dV/dt) of the intracellular
trace. The depth of the spike is proportional to MRD. Bretylium, even at a concentration of 20 mg l^{-1}, had no direct "class I" depressant effect on the cardiac
membrane.

known that in myxoedema the electrocardiogram is of low voltage and it
was a reasonable guess that the reduced metabolic rate might have
interfered in some way with the ionic pumps, so that the voltages of the
sodium and potassium batteries could have been reduced. Actual experi-
ment indicated, however, that this was not the case (Freedberg, Papp and
Vaughan Williams, 1970).

Thus was another beautiful hypothesis laid quietly to rest. Evidently alterations of thyroid state had no effect upon the resting or action potential voltages, nor was there any effect of significance on the rate of rise of the action potential. Presumably the low ECG voltage observed in myxoedema is due to some factor such as the presence of interstitial fluid or pericardial effusion. Differences in thyroid state did, however, have a very big influence on the duration of the action potential (Figs 5 and 6).

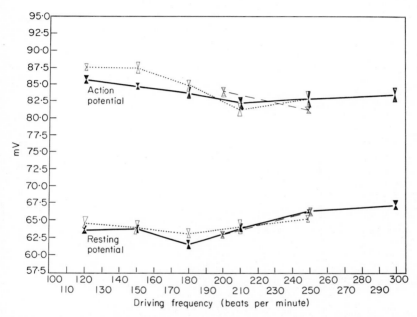

FIG. 5. Intracellularly recorded resting and action potentials of rabbit atria. To avoid errors which might be introduced by differences of spontaneous heart rate, the measurements were made in atria electrically stimulated over a wide range of frequencies. *Controls:* black triangles and solid lines. *Hyperthyroid animals:* striped triangles and dashed line. The apices of the triangles meet at the mean, and the height of each triangle equals the standard error. *Hyperthyroid:* open triangles and dotted line.

We thus seemed to have hit upon a third way in which an anti-dysrhythmic effect might be achieved, if a drug could be found, which, without being generally anti-thyroid, might nevertheless imitate the effects of hypothyroidism on cardiac muscle.

In the event, quite by chance, only a year after the investigation of the electrophysiological effects of the thyroid state, I was asked to study the mode of action of an anti-anginal drug which is not on sale in England,

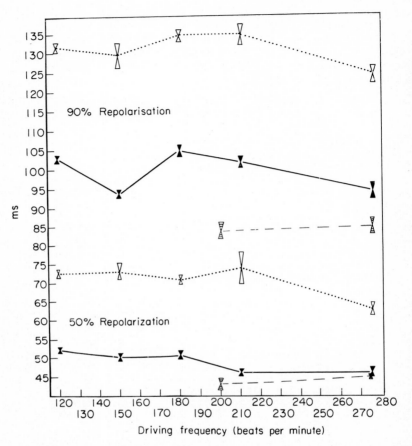

FIG. 6. Duration of action potential from peak to 90 per cent repolarization (upper curves) and to 50 per cent repolarization (lower curves). *Symbols as for Fig. 5.*

but which has been in use in Belgium, France and Germany for some years. Its name is amiodarone (Cordarone®), and its general pharmacological properties have been extensively studied by Charlier and his

Amiodarone

colleagues (1968). Our own investigations showed that this drug prolonged the cardiac action potential as did thyroidectomy (Singh and Vaughan Williams, 1970b).

It must be emphasized, however, that amiodarone is not a general antithyroid drug. It has no effect on the weight of the thyroid gland, and no signs of hypothyroidism have appeared in patients treated for prolonged periods. Amiodarone is a potent antidysrhythmic drug in animals and in man (Charlier *et al.*, 1969; Ferrero and Benabderhamane, 1972). It was of great interest subsequently to find that two of the β-adrenergic receptor blocking drugs MJ 1999 (Sotalol) and INPEA, also had this third class of antidysrhythmic action in prolonging the duration of the action potential (Singh and Vaughan Williams, 1970c; 1971a).

$$\text{X}-\!\!\!\left\langle\bigcirc\right\rangle\!\!\!-\text{CHCH}_2\text{NHCH(CH}_3)_2$$
$$\underset{\text{OH}}{|}$$

Sotalol: $X = CH_3SO_2NH-$
INPEA: $X = NO_2$

$$\underset{\text{CH}_2}{\overset{\text{CH}}{\underset{\parallel}{|}}}\!\!\overset{\text{CH}_2}{\diagup}\!\!\left\langle\bigcirc\right\rangle\!\!\overset{\text{OCH}_2\text{CHCH}_2\text{NHCH(CH}_3)_2}{\underset{\text{OH}}{|}}$$

Alprenolol

$$\underset{\underset{\text{CH}_2}{\overset{\text{CH}_2}{\underset{\diagup}{|}}}}{\overset{\text{O}}{\diagup}}\!\!\left\langle\bigcirc\right\rangle\!\!\overset{\text{OCH}_2\text{CHCH}_2\text{NHCH(CH}_3)_2}{\underset{\text{OH}}{|}}$$

Oxprenolol

To recapitulate, there are three distinct ways in which drugs may be antidysrhythmic, and several compounds have more than one kind of action. Propranolol, alprenolol (Singh and Vaughan Williams, 1970a) and oxprenolol are β-receptor blocking drugs, and are antidysrhythmic firstly because they remove sympathetic background. Secondly, at higher dosage they have class I actions as well; that is, they have a direct antidysrhythmic action by depressing the rate of rise of the action potential, as does quinidine, and incidentally are also local anaesthetics on nerve, being several times more potent than procaine. Bretylium, on the other hand, is antisympathetic without any direct class I membrane action at all. Finally there are some compounds which have a third class of action. Unlike class I drugs, which interfere with depolarization, this third class of drugs interferes with repolarization, delaying the return to the normal resting potential, and so prolonging the absolute refractory period. Interestingly enough bretylium, which has no effect on the duration of atrial action potentials, does have a class III action on ventricle.

3.4 RELEVANCE OF ACTION POTENTIAL DURATION TO ATRIAL FIBRILLATION IN MAN

From what has been said above a shortening of the action potential would automatically shorten the absolute refractory period, and should increase the probability of fibrillation. One of the simplest and most reliable methods of producing atrial fibrillation experimentally in dogs (Burn, Vaughan Williams and Walker, 1955) is to stimulate the atria electrically at high frequency during an infusion of acetylcholine, which has been shown to shorten intracellularly recorded atrial action potentials in cats (Burgen and Terroux, 1953) and rabbits (Vaughan Williams, 1958b). Fibrillation always occurs and persists after the stimulator is turned off. Anoxia (Vaughan Williams, 1970a) and halogen anaesthetics (Hauswirth, 1969) also shorten the action potential, and both are known to increase the probability of dysrhythmia. There is an association between the duration of the action potential and the incidence of fibrillation in man. Olsson, Cotoi and Varnauskas (1971) were able to record monophasic action potentials (MAPs) from patients by means of recording catheters applied by suction to the wall of the right atrium. They found, in patients who had been admitted with atrial fibrillation and who had been defibrillated electrically, that those who remained in sinus rhythm for more than three months had MAPs of normal duration, whereas all those who relapsed into fibrillation had shorter than normal MAPs. More recently Gavrilescu and Cotoi (1972) used a method similar to that of Olsson in patients with atrial fibrillation and flutter. After restoration of sinus rhythm by d.c. shock "all the patients with a right atrial monophasic action potential duration over 310 ms remained in sinus rhythm for more than three months, while four patients with a shorter right atrial MAP duration relapsed to atrial fibrillation after a period between 1 to 28 days".

3.5 A FOURTH CLASS OF ACTION?

The coronary dilator drug verapamil (iproveratril) has frequently been reported to be effective as an antidysrhythmic agent (Melville et al., 1964; Schmid and Hanna, 1967; Kaumann and Aramendia, 1968; Rodriguez-Pereira and Viana, 1968; Hanna and Schmid, 1970). Verapamil does not block the effects of isoprenaline on ventricular stroke

$$CH_3O \bigcirc \overset{\overset{\displaystyle CN}{|}}{\underset{\underset{\displaystyle CH(CH_3)_2}{|}}{C}}-CH_2CH_2\overset{\overset{\displaystyle CH_3}{|}}{N}CH_2CH_2- \bigcirc \begin{matrix} OCH_3 \\ OCH_3 \end{matrix}$$

Verapamil

volume (Ross and Jorgensen, 1967) nor on bronchial muscle (Hills, 1970), and there is other evidence that it is not a competitive antagonist of catecholamines (Nayler *et al.*, 1968; Kaumann and Aramendia, 1968). The antidysrhythmic effect of the drug cannot be attributed, therefore, to any class II or antisympathetic action, in spite of some earlier claims (Bateman, 1967). Garvey (1969) suggested that verapamil might have "quinidine-like" actions, but the electrophysiological investigations of Singh and Vaughan Williams (1972b) indicated that verapamil had no class I direct action on MRD in atrial and ventricular fibres, except at concentrations so high that contractions were abolished, and even then the effect was slight. Furthermore, the effects on the duration of the action potential were trivial, the duration to 50 per cent of repolarization (APD 50) being actually shortened, and the APD 90 being unchanged or extended by only a few milliseconds. Thus it did not appear that the antidysrhythmic action of verapamil could be explained on the basis of any of the three classes of action described above.

4 Slow inward current

Before speculating upon the possibility of a fourth class of antidysrhythmic action, it is necessary to return once more to a discussion of the cardiac action potential. As already mentioned, during the long "plateau" of the potential, especially pronounced in ventricular muscle, the mechanism by which a depolarizing "spike" of sodium current can normally enter is totally inactivated (h closed) and repolarization must proceed to about two-thirds of the resting potential before another depolarization by sodium ions would be possible. Teleologically this prolonged absolute refractoriness to sodium currents is advantageous in preventing any re-entry until the whole myocardium has been depolarized, and full synchronous activation of all contractile elements is assured.

Sodium ions are not, however, the only positive ions which can enter to carry depolarizing current. Many years ago it was shown that in the presence of increasing concentrations of quinidine the rate of rise of the action potential became slower and slower, until a "step" in it could be observed (Fig. 7). It was suggested (Vaughan Williams, 1958a) that the

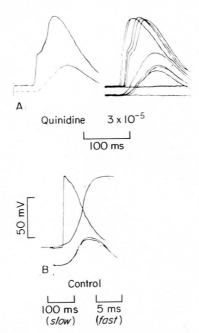

A

Quinidine 3×10^{-5}

└──┘
100 ms

50 mV

B

Control

└──┘   └──┘
100 ms   5 ms
(*slow*)   (*fast*)

FIG. 7. Effect of a high concentration of quinidine on rabbit atrial intracellular potentials. (A) *Left, upper trace:* intracellular potential. *Lower trace:* contraction. *Right:* The rate of rise became extremely slow, and ultimately a Wenckebach-type block occurred. A step developed in the upstroke of the action potential, and it is possible that the second phase of depolarizing current is carried by ions other than sodium (from Vaughan Williams, 1958a). The step almost disappeared in the action potential following the "double interval" after the missed response, which indicates that the effect of quinidine was frequency dependent; the shorter the interval between beats, the greater the effect. (B) Control tracings.

depolarizing current had two components: a fast spike, carried by sodium ions, which was reduced by quinidine; and a second, slower inward current carried by ions other than sodium, which was less affected by quinidine and was therefore revealed in the presence of the drug as a "step". This hypothesis has received considerable support from subsequent studies (Reuter, 1967; Rougier *et al.*, 1969; Besseau and Gargouil, 1969; Beeler and Reuter, 1970). Most workers in the field now agree that the fast spike of Na^+ inward depolarizing current is followed by a slower inward flow of current, carried mainly by calcium ions. There is less agreement on the extent to which the slow current (a) accounts for the plateau, or (b) is connected with the activation of contraction. It is certain, however, that the intracellular calcium concentration during diastole falls to very low levels (probably $< 10^{-7}$ M) as a result of active uptake by sarcoplasmic reticulum, and the $[Ca]_o$ to $[Ca]_i$ ratio is large enough to provide the "calcium battery" with a driving force for inward calcium current of 50–150 mV.

The substantiation of the existence of a late inward plateau current of calcium is of considerable importance in the theoretical treatment of the origin of dysrhythmias, discussed later. The inactivation of sodium current ensures that during the plateau the membrane is absolutely refractory to the recurrence of a spike carried by the fast sodium channel, but, in certain circumstances, it seems possible that a secondary depolarization carried by calcium late in the plateau, and so out of phase, might serve as an untimely stimulus to a neighbouring fibre in which excitability had been restored. If so, this might account for the antidysrhythmic action of verapamil.

There is other evidence in favour of this hypothesis: (1) verapamil in isolated cardiac muscle has an extreme negative inotropic action (Singh and Vaughan Williams, 1972b), and this would be consistent with an interference with inward calcium movements; (2) inward calcium current occurs late in the plateau, and restriction of this would also be consistent with the observed shortening of the APD 50; (3) calcium movements connected with contraction coupling are inhibited by verapamil (Fleckenstein, 1973). Graca and van Zweiten (1971) found that verapamil 5×10^{-6} M reduced ^{45}Ca uptake into isolated rabbit atria. A reduction of ^{45}Ca uptake by 5×10^{-7} M verapamil was not detectable, but it is possible, of course, that an inward Ca current capable of triggering an extrasystole might be prevented by verapamil at a concentration lower than that causing detectable changes of ^{45}Ca movements.

Whether or not inhibition of Ca current is responsible for the antidysrhythmic property of verapamil, there can be no doubt that the drug has a negative inotropic effect even in low concentration. This may be of little importance in a patient with a healthy myocardium capable of compensating for it by appropriate circulatory and autonomic reflexes, but it must be recognized as a potential danger in the clinical use of the drug.

It is of interest to note that recently Vassort and colleagues (1969) demonstrated that the late inward flow of current during the plateau is increased by adrenaline.

5 Origin of Arrhythmias

Theories concerning the aetiology of cardiac arrhythmias have a long history, and there might have been less controversy if it had been more readily appreciated that some differing explanations were not mutually exclusive. More than half a century has passed since Sir Thomas Lewis put forward his circus movement hypothesis, an idea which held the field for twenty years. The main objections to it were the following:

i. Doubt about the anatomical basis for the circus pathway. This objection now has less force since the demonstration by James (1963) of specialized conducting tissue in human atria, providing several possible fast circuits.

ii. The fact that the fibrillation induced experimentally by locally applied aconitine ceased when the ectopic focus was cooled. Here again, this objection does not apply to all experimentally induced fibrillation; for example, fibrillation precipitated by acetylcholine infusion and local electrical stimulation persists indefinitely after the ectopic stimulation is discontinued (Burn et al., 1955).

iii. High-speed cinematography and multiple surface electrical records failed to reveal any stable circuit of excitation in experimentally induced fibrillation (Prinzmetal et al., 1952).

These observations did not exclude the possibility of many small and changeable re-entry circuits, in accordance with the multiple wavelet hypothesis of Moe (1962). The basic requirements for the production of a re-entry type of fibrillation were elegantly demonstrated in a computed model by Moe et al. (1964). The model consisted of a matrix of nearly one thousand hexagonal cells, each making contact with six others (except at the borders of the matrix) in such a way that if a cell were excited it would excite its neighbours after a finite interval unless they were absolutely refractory. Excitation was followed by a short period of absolute refractoriness and successive periods of decreasing relative refractoriness (defined as a diminishing delay between excitation in a neighbour and response in a relatively refractory cell). Provided that (a) the matrix was of adequate size, (b) there was some inhomogeneity in the relative refractoriness of individual cells, (c) the refractory periods were not too long, then repetitive excitation at a point induced a fibrillatory situation in the matrix which continued to maintain multiple re-entry circuits indefinitely after the local repetitive excitation had been discontinued. The re-entry pathways were randomly distributed and no stable re-entry circuits were established, except under special circumstances such as the deletion of slots of contiguous cells. Reduction of the inhomogeneity or lengthening of the refractory periods could abort the fibrillation.

Certain analogies between this model and actual cardiac arrhythmias are obvious. Inhomogeneity in the refractory period and conduction velocity of different regions of the heart exists already (Sano et al., 1959) and is increased by anoxia, chloroform and certain drugs (Han and Moe, 1964). Pathological lesions would be likely to increase it further. An ectopic focus can be provided experimentally by aconitine or by electrical stimulation, but sources such as these are absent in man, and a very real difficulty in accepting either the re-entry hypothesis or the rival ectopic focus theory (Scherf and Schott, 1953) is that both require the existence of an abnormal stimulus from a secondary site as an initiating condition, and there is no firm evidence as to how this may be provided in man. Human arrhythmias are associated with disease processes which would be expected to depress rather than to increase excitability.

The required ectopic stimulus could, of course, be an extrasystole but this only transfers the problem to that of explaining the origin of extrasystoles. One explanation of ancient date is that "true" or coupled extrasystoles represent return re-entries across a region of intermittent block which failed to pass an outgoing action potential. This explanation was rejected by Scherf and Schott on various grounds, the most telling of which was that the coupling interval of an extrasystole is usually far longer than the conduction time of the suggested pathway. They themselves maintained that "true extrasystoles are precipitated in the ectopic centre by the preceding beat", but this fails to explain why they occur. An attractive hypothesis is that of Schamroth (1966; 1971) who suggested that there might be an independent pacemaker, as in parasystole, impulses from which were out of phase with the dominant rhythm and were usually blocked, but which could excite the heart when the rising phase of the ectopic pacemaker potential was enabled to reach threshold by summing with current spreading electrotonically from the dominant action potential across a region of block. Another explanation which could be called an "escape and reflux" (Vaughan Williams, 1971) might be considered a synthesis of Schamroth's and of the re-entry hypothesis. It is well established (Stock, 1969) that if excitation to Purkinje tissue fails, an escape beat is usually generated after an interval of between 1·0 and 1·5 seconds. If a region of complete block was surrounded by an area of intermittent block, an impulse could reach the region beyond the block by an alternative route. (If this proceeded back again across the block, it would, of course, illustrate the re-entry hypothesis.) If, however, the region of intermittent block were extended, and encroached upon the alternative route, the blocked region would fail to be excited, and might then produce an escape beat which, if it could now reflux back across the intermittently blocked area, would provide an extrasystole at the required interval. The extrasystole would thus be coupled not to the preceding beat, as suggested by Scherf and Schott, but to the one before that. Obviously if the new site continued to produce impulses at its own idiopathic frequency, it would constitute a parasystolic focus. An advantage of this hypothesis is that it explains not only the coupling of isolated extrasystoles, but also gives a reason why a train of intermittent parasystolic impulses always *starts* with a coupled beat. Some more recent theoretical work with models has suggested that an ectopic pacemaker to start off an arrhythmia may not be necessary at all, but that a spiralling type of re-entry wave could arise spontaneously from the point of contact between a conducting region and a neighbouring region in which excitation has been delayed (Krinsky et al., 1972). The difficulty with all such models is that there is no way of telling how closely they represent the real situation in man.

To what extent can it be shown that conditions comparable to those of the models exist in reality? First, in man the matrix is certainly much larger than that required by a model; moreover it is three-dimensional, whereas the model is only two-dimensional. Secondly, electron microscope studies have shown that each cardiac cell has "tight-junctions" (which are the most probable location for intercellular low-resistance pathways (Weidmann, 1966)), which join it to several others, perhaps as many as six (F.O. Simpson, personal communication). Thirdly, inhomogeneity of various parameters has been demonstrated, as already mentioned. Fourthly, the greater probability of dysrhythmias associated with a short action potential has been described in man, whereas in hypothyroidism rarity of dysrhythmias is associated with a long one. Finally, sources of ectopic activation are a common feature of numerous pathological cardiac states, and the importance of parasystolic pacemakers in the aetiology of many kinds of human dysrhythmia has been emphasized by Schamroth (1971).

How, then, may the three classes of antidysrhythmic action described above be related to the theoretical considerations concerning the cellular basis of cardiac dysrhythmias? The class II (antisympathetic) action can remove or retard parasystolic pacemaking sources activated by excessive sympathetic activity or by circulating catecholamines. Antisympathetic action may also prevent some direct action of catecholamines on the membrane, altering ionic conductances in such a way as to predispose to conduction abnormalities (Hauswirth et al., 1968; 1972), although the technique by which this evidence was obtained has met some criticism (Johnson and Lieberman, 1971). The third class of action, by prolonging the cardiac action potential, would push the absolute refractory period beyond the limiting value. Finally, the first class of action would directly impede cell-to-cell conduction at a high frequency. Thus the analysis of antidysrhythmic action into the three classes described above does fit rather well theories concerning the cellular basis of cardiac dysrhythmias.

6 Paradoxical evidence

The above classification of antidysrhythmic actions and its application to model requirements for fibrillation may appear almost too neat and tidy, and attention must now be paid to some inconvenient observations which seem at first sight to be out of line. For example it has been reported that diphenylhydantoin (DPH, phenytoin, dilantin®) 10 mg kg^{-1} i.v *accelerated* conduction from the atrium to the bundle of His in un-anaesthetized dogs (Rosati *et al.*, 1967), although conduction velocity was slowed elsewhere in the heart. It has been repeatedly stressed, however, that although there seems good reason to include DPH with drugs having class I actions on the cardiac membrane, depressing MRD, this is not to suggest that all such compounds have identical actions in the *whole animal*. On the contrary, there are many important differences in absorption and distribution, actions on the CNS and peripheral nerves, atropine-like actions etc. Diphenylhydantoin is an anti-epileptic drug, and was only introduced as an antidysrhythmic one on the rather fanciful basis that drugs capable of controlling "abnormal rhythm" in the brain might also do the same in the heart. Thus it is quite possible that the shortening of A–V conduction time by DPH may be secondary to noradrenaline release from sympathetic nerve endings as a result of an action of the drug on the CNS or on peripheral nerves. In support of this view is the finding of Bigger, Strauss and Hoffman (1968) that diphenyl-hydantoin did *not* accelerate A–V conduction "in preparations from rabbits given reserpine for two days before sacrifice". The accelerating effect was also attenuated by propranolol. Furthermore, Sasyniuk and Dresel (1968) found only a slowing, never an acceleration, of A–V conduction in *isolated* blood-perfused hearts. Thus the acceleration of A–V conduction by DPH in whole animals can be regarded as a side effect, which, except in certain circumstances (see below), might actually increase the probability of dysrhythmia. Similarly, there is no rational basis for considering that the shortening of the action potential by lignocaine and DPH contributes to their antidysrhythmic action. On the contrary, such an effect might be expected to be disadvantageous, increasing the probability of re-entry.

In certain clinical situations, however, A–V conduction or normal impulse formation may be impaired, resulting in an increase of inhomogeneity of current distribution and a break-up of the action potential wave front. Partial block carries the risk of escape beats occurring out of phase, and in these circumstances, especially if there is bradycardia, speeding up of A–V conduction and impulse formation in pacemaking tissue by atropine or isoprenaline could be beneficial, in spite of the risk of activating ectopic pacemakers as well. The "antidysrhythmic" action of atropine which is sometimes observed could, therefore, partly be attributed to an action of this kind, improved conduction leading to increased synchronicity. Alternatively, if there is high vagal activity, the acetylcholine released would shorten atrial action potentials, and atropine could be antidysrhythmic by restoring the phase of repolarization to its normal duration (i.e. atropine has class III activity if vagal tone is high). Obviously the interpretation of apparent anomalies of this kind must depend on knowledge of conduction defects and other abnormalities in each individual case.

Finally some explanation must be found for the well-known paradox that sometimes exhibition of antidysrhythmic drugs with class I actions, especially quinidine, may actually appear to precipitate a dysrhythmia. Here, again, the interpretation requires knowledge of individual circumstances. But one might speculate that in a situation in which partial conduction defects already exist, and have led to considerable inhomogeneity in distribution of the wavefront, further depression of conduction in abnormal tissue could lead to completion of a return circuit, so that re-entry now occurred. The solution would not be to stop administering the drug, but to increase it, so that the abnormal return pathway would also be blocked.

7 New antidysrhythmic drugs

The foregoing account represents an attempt to describe some hard facts about the accurately measurable properties which known antidysrhythmic drugs actually possess, and to classify them in such a way that a rational and coherent explanation can be given of their probable mode of action. It is fully recognized that other authors have come to different conclusions. For this reason considerable attention has been paid to presenting in some detail the experimental work upon which differing views have been based, and to citing the sources liberally, so that the interested reader may judge for himself where, in the scales of probability, the balance of evidence lies. The crucial issue is whether the analysis presented permits predictions to be made as to the antidysrhythmic efficacy of new compounds. If a new drug is found in pharmacological tests to reduce MRD in cardiac muscle, or to be antisympathetic, or to prolong the duration of the action potential, or to reduce Ca influx, will it prove to be an antidysrhythmic agent in man?

Lignocaine is an extremely useful drug, and since it is rapidly metabolized to inactive products in the liver, it is also very safe. On the other hand the very fact that it disappears so quickly from the portal circulation carries the requirement that it be administered parenterally. There is, therefore, a need for a drug with a class I action on the cardiac membrane, which is rapidly absorbed orally and which has a reasonably long duration of action. Two compounds have recently been found with these properties, L7810, a decahydroquinoline derivative (Bagwell Polster and Vaughan Williams, 1973), and mexitelline (Kö 1173) (Allen *et al.*, 1970; Singh and Vaughan Williams, 1972a). The latter has been submitted to clinical trial, and has indeed proved to be antidysrhythmic, with an efficacy comparable with that of lignocaine (Clark *et al.*, 1973; Campbell *et al.*, 1973).

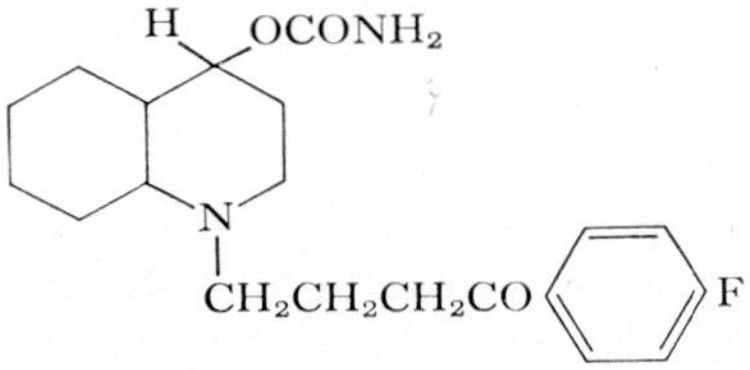

L 7810

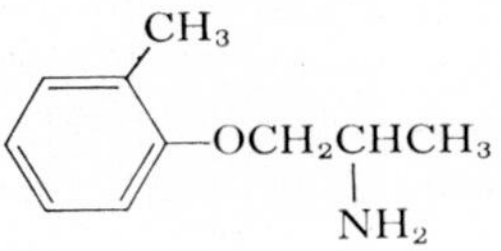

Mexitelline

Amiodarone, originally introduced as an antianginal drug, should also be antidysrhythmic, because it has some class I and class II actions, and a very pronounced class III action upon prolonged administration. Here, again, this drug has been shown to be antidysrhythmic in man (Ferrero and Benabderhamane, 1972), and is especially effective in maintaining in sinus rhythm patients who had been treated by d.c. shock for atrial fibrillation (S. B. Olsson, personal communication). Prolonged treatment of animals with oxyfedrine, another antianginal drug, also delayed repolarization in cardiac muscle (Polster and Vaughan Williams, 1972), and the prediction would be that this compound, too, could be antidysrhythmic.

8 Conclusions

Even if, for the sake of argument, the classification of antidysrhythmic drugs outlined above, and its relevance to models of dysrhythmias, were accepted, the physician might still wonder whether he is any nearer, in

practical terms, to a rational approach to the treatment of clinically
encountered abnormalities of cardiac rhythm. The concluding para-
graphs are addressed to this question.

Clearly the problem of treatment is greatly simplified if a dysrhythmia
is primary and there is no evidence of myocardial degeneration or

CH$_3$O

$$\text{—CCH}_2\text{CH}_2\text{NHCHCH—}$$
O   CH$_3$ OH

Oxyfedrine

cardiac vascular disease. In a post-menopausal woman, for example,
whose tachycardia is largely caused or exacerbated by anxiety, exhibition
of a class II antisympathetic drug would be rational therapy, and a
β-receptor blocker provides adequate control in doses too small to present any danger. The same applies to other stress induced dysrhythmias,
as during induction of anaesthesia (Payne and Senfield, 1964) or such
occupations as skiing, flying, driving, public speaking etc. (Eliasch et al.,
1967; Imhof et al., 1969; Taggart et al., 1969; Somerville et al., 1971). In
such circumstances the choice of any particular β-blocking drug is probably of little importance.

Atrial fibrillation can usually be corrected by d.c. shock, but main-
tenance in sinus rhythm remains a problem. Patients who relapse into
fibrillation have shorter than normal action potentials, and exhibition of a
drug with a class III action, prolonging the duration of the action potential, would be appropriate. Amiodarone and oxyfedrine both have such
an action on prolonged treatment.

When a dysrhythmia is a manifestation of serious cardiac disease,
however, control is more difficult and dangerous, and even though
correction of the abnormal rhythm may prolong life, it does not, of
course, remove the underlying pathology. After cardiac infarction
dysrhythmias occur in 90 per cent or more of patients (Julian et al., 1964).
Factors increasing the probability of re-entry are the shortening of action
potentials in hypoxic fibres, and inhomogeneity of conduction pathways
through and around damaged areas. In addition, the level of circulating
catecholamines is extremely high (Valori et al., 1967) and has been correlated with the incidence of rhythm abnormalities. In these circumstances
also, therefore, exhibition of a β-blocker would be rational therapy, but
brings with it the danger than an ailing myocardium deprived of its
sympathetic drive may fail altogether. What is needed is a drug which

could block receptors mediating chronotropic effects without blocking those mediating inotropic effects, but no such compound is yet available. In its absence, extreme caution is necessary, so that a level of blockade is selected which eliminates the excessive adrenergic stimulation facilitating the development of dysrhythmias, but which is not so complete that inotropic drive is endangered. The choice of drug may be important, and in this context three considerations are relevant.

1. It has been suggested that β-receptor blocking drugs which have some partial agonist (sympathomimetic) activity of their own may be preferable (e.g. alprenolol, Åblad et al., 1967). The logic of this is not apparent, however. Why should the activity of a partial agonist be preferable to that of noradrenaline and adrenaline, themselves the natural transmitters? If agonist activity is required, it should be sufficient to reduce the degree of blockade.

2. Some β-blockers have class I activity as well (notably propranolol, alprenolol and oxprenolol (Morales-Aguilerá and Vaughan Williams, 1965; Vaughan Williams and Papp, 1970; Singh and Vaughan Williams, 1970a), and it has been suggested that this "nonspecific" depressant activity may be associated with a negative inotropic action (Gent et al., 1970). If this were so, practolol and pindolol (LB 46) would be advantageous (Singh and Vaughan Williams, 1971a), but no satisfactory evidence is available that the liability of β-blockers to precipitate failure is in fact related to any direct negative inotropic action.

OCH₂CHCH₂NHCH(CH₃)₂

OH

NHCOCH₃

Practolol

OCH₂CHCH₂NHCH(CH₃)₂

OH

N
H

Pindolol

3. Some β-receptor blocking drugs are more active in blocking peripheral receptors (mediating vasodilatation in the limbs) than in blocking cardiac receptors. Among such drugs are pindolol and propranolol, and the compounds with substituents at position 2 of the ring, alprenolol and oxprenolol (Vaughan Williams et al., 1973). These compounds, against a background of circulating catecholamines, are actually *hyper*tensive (Nakano and Kusakari, 1965; Kayaalp and Kiran, 1966; Yamamoto and Sekiya, 1972). It is possible, therefore, that such β-blockers could, on the background of a high level of circulating catecholamines, cause a rise in peripheral resistance which could throw an additional load on the

myocardium. If this is so, a cardioselective β-receptor blocking drug, such as practolol, would have an advantage. One of the features conferring cardioselectivity is substitution on position 4 of the ring (Vaughan Williams *et al.*, 1973; Bagwell and Vaughan Williams, 1973), and doubtless new compounds even more cardioselective than practolol will eventually be available.

Which, if any, of the above considerations is important will have to be determined by further research.

Diminution of sympathetic background removes only one of the factors increasing the probability of dysrhythmias, and when this is insufficient recourse to a drug with a class I action is necessary. If exhibition of such compounds (lignocaine, procainamide, diphenyl-hydantoin, quinidine) is still ineffective, an obvious precaution is to measure the serum potassium level, and if this is low, to correct it. Theoretically, it would seem justifiable to raise the serum potassium above normal, in order to increase the efficacy of the drug, but here again further research is required to determine how far this would be a safe procedure.

Finally, in the future, it is probable that drugs with an acute class III action will become available. At present the only drugs with such an acute action, INPEA and sotalol, are also β-blockers, and the class III action would be accompanied by further β-blockade. Amiodarone and oxyfedrine require prolonged administration to produce this effect.

In conclusion, it is apparent that so far there is no established procedure, authenticated by experimental evidence, the progressive application of which would ensure the optimum utilization of currently available drugs to correct dysrhythmias in gravely ill patients. On the other hand, a great deal is known of the electrophysiological and pharmacological properties of the individual compounds, so that the research from which such a procedure may emerge can at least now be planned on a rational basis.

References

Åblad, B., Brogård, M. and Ek, L. (1967). Pharmacological properties of H56/28—a β-adrenergic receptor antagonist. *Acta Pharmacol. Toxicol.* 25, Suppl. 2, 9.

Allen, J. D., Kofi Ekue, J. M., Shanks, R. G. and Zaidi, S. A. (1970). The effect on experimental cardiac arrhythmias of a new anticonvulsant agent, Kö 1173, and its comparison with phenytoin and procainamide. *Brit. J. Pharmacol. Chemother.* 39, 183.

Bagwell, E. E., Polster, P. and Vaughan Williams, E. M. (1973). The effects on cardiac muscle and nerve of a fluorinated decahydroquinoline derivative, L 7810, rapidly absorbed after oral administration. *Brit. J. Pharmacol. Chemother.* 43, 183.

Bagwell, E. E. and Vaughan Williams, E. M. (1973). Further studies regarding the structure activity relationships of β-adrenoceptor antagonists. *Brit. J. Pharmacol. Chemother.* **48**, 686.

Bassett, A. L. and Hoffman, B. F. (1971). Anti-arrhythmic drugs: electrophysiological actions. *Ann. Rev. Pharmacol.* **11**, 143.

Bateman, F. J. A. (1967). What is a β-blocker? *Lancet*, **ii**, 418.

Beeler, G. W. and Reuter, H. (1970). Membrane calcium current in ventricular myocardial fibres. *J. Physiol. (London)*, **207**, 191.

Besseau, A. and Gargouïl, Y. M. (1969). Ionic currents in rat ventricular heart fibres: voltage-clamp experiments using double sucrose-gap technique. *J. Physiol. (London)*, **204**, 95.

Bigger, J. T. and Mandel, W. J. (1970). Effect of lidocaine on the electrophysiological properties of ventricular muscle and Purkinje fibres. *J. Clin. Invest.* **49**, 63.

Bigger, J. T., Strauss, H. C. and Hoffman, B. F. (1968). Effects of diphenylhydantoin on atrioventricular conduction. *Fed. Proc.* **27**, 406.

Burgen, A. S. V. and Terroux, Kathleen, G. (1953). On the negative inotropic effect in the cat's auricle. *J. Physiol. (London)*, **120**, 449.

Burn, J. H., Vaughan Williams, E. M. and Walker, J. M. (1955). The effects of acetylcholine in the heart–lung preparation including the production of auricular fibrillation. *J. Physiol. (London)*, **128**, 277.

Campbell, N., Kelly, J., Strong, J., Shanks, R. G. and Pantridge, J. P. (1973). Effects of Kö 1173 on ventricular arrhythmias. *Brit. Heart J.* **35**, 559.

Charlier, R., Deltour, G., Baudine, A. and Chaillet, F. (1968). Pharmacology of amiodarone, an anti-anginal drug with a new biological profile. *Arzneimittelforsch.* **18**, 1408.

Charlier, R., Delaunois, G., Bauthier, J. and Deltour, G. (1969). Dans la série des benzofurannes. XL. Propriétés antiarrhythmiques de l'amiodarone. *Cardiologia*, **54**, 83.

Clark, R. A. Talbot, R. G., Nimmo, J., Prescott, L. F. and Julian, D. G. (1973). Kö 1173—an effective new antidysrhythmic drug. *Brit. Heart J.* **35**, 558.

Davis, L. D. and Temte, J. V. (1969). Electrophysiological actions of lidocaine on canine ventricular muscle and Purkinje fibre. *Circulation Res.* **24**, 639.

Dohadwalla, A. N., Freedberg, A. S. and Vaughan Williams, E. M. (1969). The relevance of β-receptor blockade to ouabain-induced cardiac arrhythmias. *Brit. J. Pharmacol. Chemother.* **36**, 257.

Eliasch, H., Rosen, A. and Scott, H. M. (1967). Systemic circulatory response to stress of simulated flight and to physical exercise before and after propranolol blockade. *Brit. Heart J.* **29**, 671.

Ferrero, C. and Benabderhamane, M. (1972). Terapia medica del flutter atriale. *Giorn. Ital. Card.* **2**, 186.

Fleckenstein, A. (1973). Drug induced changes in cardiac energy. Conference on the Myocardium, Canberra. In press.

Freedberg, A. S., Papp, J. Gy. and Vaughan Williams, E. M. (1970). The effect of altered thyroid state on atrial intracellular potentials. *J. Physiol. (London)*, **207**, 357.

Garvey, H. L. (1969). The mechanism of action of verapamil on the sinus and AV nodes. *Europ. J. Pharmacol.* **8**, 159.

Gavrilescu, S. and Cotoi, S. (1972). Monophasic action potential of right human atrium during atrial flutter and after conversion to sinus rhythm. *Brit. Heart J.* **34**, 396.

Gent, G., Davis, T. C. and McDonald, A. (1970). Practolol in treatment of supraventricular cardiac dysrhythmias. *Brit. Med. J.* **i**, 533.

Goodford, P. J. and Vaughan Williams, E. M. (1962). Intracellular Na and K concentrations of rabbit atria, in relation to the action of quinidine. *J. Physiol. (London)*, **160**, 483.

Graça, A. S. and van Zwieten, P. A. (1971). The influence of iproveratril on calcium movements in isolated heart muscle. *Europ. J. Pharmacol.* **15**, 137.

Han, J. and Moe, G. K. (1964). Non-uniform recovery of excitability in ventricular muscle. *Circulation Res.* **14**, 44.

Hanna, C. and Schmid, J. R. (1970). Antiarrhythmic actions of coronary vasodilator agents papaverine, dioxyline and verapamil. *Arch. Int. Pharmacodyn. Ther.* **185**, 228.

Hauswirth, O. (1969). Effects of halothane on single atrial, ventricular and Purkinje fibres. *Circulation Res.* **24**, 745.

Hauswirth, O., Noble, D. and Tsien, R. W. (1968). Adrenaline: mechanism of action on the pacemaker potential in cardiac Purkinje fibers. *Science*, **162**, 916.

Hauswirth, O., Noble, D. and Tsien, R. W. (1972). Separation of the pace-maker and plateau components of delayed rectification in cardiac Purkinje fibres. *J. Physiol. (London)*, **225**, 211.

Hills, E. A. (1970). Iproveratril and bronchial asthma. *Brit. J. Clin. Practice*, **24**, 116.

Hodgkin, A. L. (1958). Ionic movements and electrical activity in giant nerve fibres. *Proc. Roy. Soc. B.*, **148**, 1.

Imhof, P. R., Blatter, K., Fucella, L. M. and Turri, M. (1969). Beta-blockade and emotional tachycardia: radio telemetric investigations in ski jumpers. *J. Appl. Physiol.* **27**, 366.

James, T. N. (1963). The connecting pathways between the sinus node and A–V node and between the right and left atrium in the human heart. *Amer. Heart J.* **66**, 498.

Johnson, E. A. and Lieberman, M. (1971). Heart: excitation and contraction. *Ann. Res. Physiol.* **33**, 479.

Julian, D. G., Valentine, P. A. and Miller, G. G. (1964). Disturbances of rate, rhythm and conduction in acute myocardial infarction. *Amer. J. Med.* **37**, 915.

Kaumann, A. J. and Aramendia, P. (1968). Prevention of ventricular fibrillation induced by coronary ligation. *J. Pharmacol. Exp. Ther.* **164**, 326.

Kayaalp, S. O. and Kiran, B. K. (1966). Mechanism of a sympathomimetic action of propranolol in dogs. *Brit. J. Pharmacol. Chemother.* **28**, 15.

Krinsky, V. I., Pertsov, A. M. and Reshetilov, A. N. (1972). Wave-sources and cardiac arrhythmias. IV Internat. Biophys. Cong. E. XIV 95/3. In press.

Melville, K. I., Shister, H. E. and Huq, S. (1964). Iproveratril: experimental data on coronary dilatation and antiarrhythmic action. *Canad. Med. Ass. J.* **90**, 761.

Méndez, C., Acevez, J. and Méndez, R. (1961). The anti-adrenergic action of digitalis on the refractory period of the A–V transmission system. *J. Pharmacol. Exp. Ther.* **131**, 199.

Moe, G. K. (1962). On the multiple wavelet hypothesis of atrial fibrillation. *Arch. Int. Pharmacodyn. Ther.* **140**, 183.

Moe, G. K., Rheinboldt, W. C. and Abildskov, J. A. (1964). A computer model of atrial fibrillation. *Amer. Heart. J.* **67**, 200.

Morales-Aguilerá, A. and Vaughan Williams, E. M. (1965). The effects on cardiac muscle of β-receptor antagonists in relation to their activity as local anaesthetics. *Brit. J. Pharmacol.* **24**, 332.

Nakano, J. and Kusakari, T. (1965). Effect of propranolol on the peripheral circulation. *Proc. Soc. Exp. Biol. Med.* **120**, 516.

Nayler, W. G., McInnes, I., Swann, J. B., Price, J. M., Carson, V., Race, D. and Lowe, T. E. (1968). Some effects of iproveratril (Isoptin) on the cardiovascular system. *J. Pharmacol. Exp. Ther.* **161**, 247.

Olsson, S. B., Cotoi, S. and Varnauskas, E. (1971). Monophasic action potential and sinus rhythm stability after conversion of atrial fibrillation. *Acta Med. Scand.* **190**, 381.

Pamintuan, J. C., Dreifus, L. S. and Watanabe, Y. (1970). Comparative mechanisms of antiarrhythmic drugs. *Amer. J. Cardiol.* **26**, 512.

Papp, J. Gy. and Vaughan Williams, E. M. (1969). The effect of bretylium on intracellular cardiac action potentials in relation to its anti-arrhythmic and local anaesthetic activity. *Brit. J. Pharmacol. Chemother.* **37**, 380.

Payne, J. P. and Senfield, R. M. (1964). Pronethalol in the treatment of ventricular arrhythmias during anaesthesia. *Brit. Med. J.* **i**, 603.

Polster, P. and Vaughan Williams, E. M. (1972). The effect of prolonged treatment with oxyfedrine on intracellular potentials and on other features of cardiac function in rabbits and guinea-pigs. *Brit. J. Pharmacol. Chemother.* **47**, 187.

Prinzmetal, M., Corday, E., Brill, I. C., Oblath, R. W. and Kruger, H. E. (1952). "The Auricular Arrhythmias". Charles C. Thomas, Springfield.

Reuter, H. (1967). The dependence of slow inward current in Purkinje fibres on the extracellular calcium concentration. *J. Physiol. (London)*, **192**, 479.

Rissanen, V. T. (1970). Occurrence of coronary occlusion in cases of coronary death and accidental death. *Advan. Cardiol.* **4**, 99.

Rodrigues-Pereira, E. and Viana, A. P. (1968). The actions of verapamil on experimental arrhythmias. *Arzneimittel Forschung*, **18**, 175.

Rosati, R. A., Alexander, J. A., Schaal, S. F. and Wallace, A. G. (1967). Influence of diphenylhydantoin on electrophysiological properties of canine heart. *Circulation Res.* **21**, 757.

Ross. G. and Jorgensen, C. R. (1967). Cardiovascular actions of iproveratril. *J. Pharmacol. Exp. Ther.* **158**, 504.

Rougier, O., Vassort, G., Garnier, D., Gargouïl, Y. M. and Coraboeuf, E. (1969). Existence and role of a slow inward current during the frog atrial action potential. *Pfluegers Arch. Gesamte Physiol. Menschen Tiere*, **308**, 91.

Sano, T., Takayama, N. and Shimamoto, T. (1959). Directional difference of conduction velocity in the cardiac ventricular syncytium studied by microelectrodes. *Circulation Res.* **7**, 262.

Sasyniuk, B. I. and Dresel, P. E. (1968). The effect of diphenylhydantoin on conduction in isolated, blood perfused hearts. *J. Pharmacol. Exp. Ther.* **161**, 191.

Schamroth, L. (1966). Genesis and evolution of ectopic ventricular rhythm. *Brit. Heart J.* **28**, 244.

Schamroth, L. (1971). The physiological basis of ectopic ventricular rhythm: a unifying concept. *South Afr. Med. J. Supplement*, 3.

Scherf, D. and Schott, A. (1953). "Extrasystoles and Allied Arrhythmias". Heineman, London.

Schmid, J. R. and Hanna, C. (1967). A comparison of the antiarrhythmic actions of two new synthetic compounds, iproveratril and MJ 1999, with quinidine and pronethalol. *J. Pharmacol. Exp. Ther.* **156**, 331.

Singh, B. N. and Vaughan Williams, E. M. (1970a). Local anaesthetic and anti-arrhythmic actions of alprenolol relative to its effect on intracellular potentials and other properties of isolated cardiac muscle. *Brit. J. Pharmacol. Chemother.* **38**, 749.

Singh, B. N. and Vaughan Williams, E. M. (1970b). The effect of amiodarone, a new anti-anginal drug on cardiac muscle. *Brit. J. Pharmacol. Chemother.* **39**, 657.

Singh, B. N. and Vaughan Williams, E. M. (1970c). A third class of anti-arrhythmic action. Effects on atrial and ventricular intracellular potentials, and other pharmacological actions on cardiac muscle, of MJ 1999 and AH 3474. *Brit. J. Pharmacol. Chemother.* **39**, 675.

Singh, B. N. and Vaughan Williams, E. M. (1971a). The effect on cardiac muscle of the β-adrenoceptor blocking drugs INPEA and LB 46 in relation to their local anaesthetic action on nerve. *Brit. J. Pharmacol. Chemother.* **43**, 10.

Singh, B. N. and Vaughan Williams, E. M. (1971b). The effect of altering potassium concentration on the action of lidocaine and diphenylhydantoin on rabbit atrial and ventricular muscle. *Circulation Res.* **29**, 286.

Singh, B. N. and Vaughan Williams, E. M. (1972a). Investigations of the mode of action of a new antidysrhythmic drug, Kö 1173. *Brit. J. Pharmacol. Chemother.* **44**, 1.

Singh, B. N. and Vaughan Williams, E. M. (1972b). A fourth class of antidysrhythmic action? Effect of verapamil on ouabain toxicity, on atrial and ventricular intracellular potentials, and on other features of cardiac function. *Cardiovasc. Res.* **6**, 109.

Somerville, W., Taggart, P. and Carruthers, M. (1971). Addressing a medical meeting: effect on heart rate, electrocardiogram, plasma catecholamines, free fatty acids and triglycerides. *Brit. Heart J.* **33**, 608.

Stock, J. P. P. (1969). "Diagnosis and Treatment of Cardiac Arrhythmias". Butterworths, London.

Taggart, P., Gibbons, D. and Somerville, W. (1969). Some effects of motor car driving on the normal and abnormal heart. *Brit. Med. J.* **4**, 130.

Valori, C., Thomas, M. and Shillingford, J. P. (1967). Urinary excretion of free noradrenaline and adrenaline following acute myocardial infarction. *Lancet*, **i**, 127.

Vassort, G., Rougier, O., Garnier, D., Sauviat, M. P., Coraboeuf, E. and Gargouïl, Y. M. (1969). Effects of adrenaline of membrane inward currents during the cardiac action potential. *Pfluegers Arch. Gesamte Physiol. Menschen Tiere.* **309**, 70.

Vaughan Williams, E. M. (1958a). The mode of action of quinidine in isolated rabbit atria interpreted from intracellular records. *Brit. J. Pharmacol. Chemother.* **13**, 276.

Vaughan Williams, E. M. (1958b). Some observations concerning the mode of action of acetylcholine on isolated rabbit atria. *J. Physiol. (London)*, **140**, 327.

Vaughan Williams, E. M. (1961). The action of quinidine, acetylcholine and anaphylaxis interpreted from simultaneous records of contractions and intracellular potentials in the heart. Scientific basis of Medicine, *Annual Reviews*, 302–323. The Athlone Press, London.

Vaughan Williams, E. M. (1970a). Experimental basis for the choice of an anti-arrhythmic drug. *Advan. Cardiol.* **4**, 275

Vaughan Williams, E. M. (1970b). Classification of anti-arrhythmic drugs. *In*

"Symposium on Cardiac Arrhythmias" (Eds E. Sandøe, E. Flensted-Jensen and K. H. Olesen), pp. 449–472. AB Astra, Södertälje, Sweden.

Vaughan Williams, E. M. (1971). Electrophysiology of cardiac arrhythmias. *In* Symposium on "Lidocaine in the Treatment of Ventricular Arrhythmias" (Eds D. B. Scott and D. G. Julian). Livingstone, Edinburgh.

Vaughan Williams, E. M. and Papp, J. Gy. (1970). The effect of oxprenolol on cardiac intracellular potentials in relation to its anti-arrhythmic, local anaesthetic and other properties. *Postgrad. Med. J. Nov. Suppl.* 22.

Vaughan Williams, E. M. and Sekiya, A. (1963). Prevention of arrhythmias due to cardiac glycosides by block of β-sympathetic receptors. *Lancet*, **i**, 420.

Vaughan Williams, E. M., Bagwell, E. E. and Singh, B. N. (1973). Cardiospecificity of β-receptor blockade. A comparison of the relative potencies on cardiac and peripheral β-adrenoceptors of propranolol, of practolol and its ortho-substituted isomer, and of oxprenolol and its para-substituted isomer. *Cardiovasc. Res.* **7**, 226.

Weidmann, S. (1966). The diffusion of radiopotassium across intercalated disks of mammalian cardiac muscle. *J. Physiol. (London)*, **187**, 323.

Yamamoto, J. and Sekiya, A. (1972). Further studies on the pressor action of propranolol in the rat. *Arch. Int. Pharmacodyn. Ther.* **198**, 347.

Pharmacological Approaches to the Therapy of Angina

J. R. PARRATT, BPharm, MSc, PhD, FPS

Department of Physiology and Pharmacology, Royal College, University of Strathclyde, Glasgow

1   Introduction

There are several basic difficulties for the industrial pharmacologist who has been assigned the task of developing or examining new drugs for potential antianginal activity, or for initiating research in this field. There is no suitable animal model for angina pectoris and the animals he does use are more often than not anaesthetized and have essentially normal coronary arteries. There appear to be two main lines of approach to the problem. Firstly, to work back from clinical data available regarding the detailed haemodynamic changes that take place in angina; it is only in the

103

last few years that these have been adequately evaluated. Secondly, to re-examine the pharmacology of those drugs that have been clearly demonstrated to be effective in this condition. Despite the extensive pharmacological and clinical evaluation of a large number of varied drugs (admirably summarized, for example, by Charlier, 1961, and 1971) there are probably only two drugs, or groups of drugs, which most investigators would agree are of real clinical value, nitroglycerin and the β-adreno-ceptor blocking agents.

Until about ten years ago the approach of most pharmacologists to the problem of the therapy of angina was that of producing specific, highly effective, orally active, coronary vasodilator drugs. This approach met with considerable pharmacological success and some of these drugs (particularly those that inhibit the uptake or degradation of adenosine) have been used as research tools for the study of basic problems of control of the coronary circulation. The pharmacological and clinical effects of such coronary vasodilator drugs have been reviewed recently by Parratt (1969a) and by Charlier (1971). Despite the great effectiveness of these drugs in increasing blood flow through the normal myocardium, double-blind studies have invariably shown that coronary vasodilators do not consistently alleviate anginal symptoms (see Aronow, 1972, and Charlier, 1971). The reason for this is not difficult to understand. In normal individuals increased myocardial oxygen demand is matched by a corresponding increase in myocardial blood flow. This capacity for increasing the blood supply to meet increased myocardial oxygen demands is limited in patients with sclerotic vessels. It is likely that in such patients, even at rest, there is considerable arteriolar vasodilatation in order to compensate for lumen obstruction in the main supplying arteries. This would mean that arteriolar reserve for conditions of stress is severely limited. If it is true that, in order to maintain a normal flow to the myocardial cells the majority of arterioles are dilated, then there seems little validity for giving vasodilator drugs that act on this segment of the vascular bed. Indeed, if there were any arteriolar reserve in these patients, one would expect that the reduction in myocardial oxygen tension that would result from increased cardiac work would itself act as a potent stimulus for vaso-dilatation. This hypoxia-induced vasodilatation is probably maximal during an attack of angina and an increased cellular supply of oxygen can only be achieved by the increased extraction of oxygen from blood (Gor-lin, 1960). This is limited since myocardial oxygen extraction is considerable even under normal, resting, conditions. The implication of this for the pharmacologist is that animal models which allow only measurement of total coronary flow are unlikely to be relevant to the problem of screening drugs for antianginal activity.

2   The fundamental problem: imbalance between myocardial oxygen supply and demand

The fundamental problem for the patient with angina is an imbalance between myocardial oxygen requirements and supply. This imbalance leads to acute, reversible, ventricular failure and to pain. When myocardial oxygen demands are increased (as, for example, during exercise or excitement) the supply of oxygen to the tissues is insufficient to meet the new requirements. The reason for this is some increase in resistance to flow through the coronary vessels. Until recently it has been assumed that this inadequacy of flow is due primarily to atherosclerotic changes in the coronary vessels leading to a restricted lumen. This is undoubtedly true but there are indications that this may not be the only factor involved.

Severe coronary atherosclerosis only rarely leads to symptoms of angina. In an unselected group of 430 autopsied patients Allison and his colleagues (Allison *et al.*, 1963) found evidence of coronary artery disease in 82 per cent although less than 10 per cent had a history of angina. A majority of patients with severe coronary artery disease (as documented by post-mortem coronary angiograms) did not have a history of angina pectoris (Allison *et al.*, 1963; Hershberg, 1971).

Classical angina pectoris occurs not uncommonly in patients with no demonstrable coronary atherosclerotic lesions. In various studies, normal coronary angiograms have been found in 9–36 per cent of all anginal patients examined (Aronow, 1973). This may of course be partially due to inadequacies in the technique of coronary angiography, in certain hands, to detect significant coronary stenosis, particularly in small vessels. However, published reports are now too numerous for this to be the whole explanation (e.g. recent reports by Dwyer *et al.*, 1969; Christian and Botti, 1972; Neill *et al.*, 1972; Arbogast and Bourassa, 1973; Bemiller *et al.*, 1973; MacAlpine *et al.*, 1973; Oliva *et al.*, 1973, and reviewed by Hellstrom, 1973). There appear to be two possible mechanisms for this type of angina: (*a*) an abnormal affinity of haemoglobin for oxygen (Eliot and Bratt, 1969); (*b*) a reflex coronary artery (or arteriolar) spasm (Hellstrom, 1973).

2.1   CORONARY SPASM

The concept of reflex coronary spasm is not new and was mentioned, for example, by Osler in 1897. It has been recognized that the frequency of attacks in susceptible individuals may be increased following the ingestion of food and Nigaglioni *et al.* (1963) described an individual who developed anginal pain as a result of distending the stomach with air.

Myocardial infarction in the absence of coronary atherosclerosis, and apparently resulting from severe spasm of the left circumflex artery, has also recently been described (Cheng *et al.*, 1972). In animals, Kaverina (1965) has been largely instrumental for drawing attention to the importance of reflex activity from the viscera in the development of acute coronary insufficiency and recently Moore and I (Moore and Parratt, 1974) have found that distending the small intestine, or bladder, with air can on occasions decrease myocardial blood flow in anaesthetized cats, despite elevations of systemic arterial pressure. Two such experiments are illustrated in Figs 1 and 2. It is the author's view that there is now

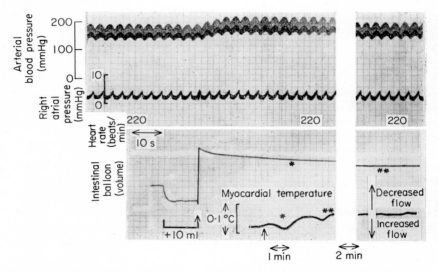

FIG. 1. Evidence of coronary vasoconstriction. The effect of increasing the pressure within a balloon inserted into the lumen of an anaesthetized cat on, from above, arterial blood pressure (mmHg), right atrial pressure (mmHg), intestinal volume, and myocardial temperature recorded from an implanted heated thermocouple. Increasing the pressure within the balloon resulted in an increase in systemic pressure of 20 to 25 mmHg and an immediate increase in myocardial blood flow. After 2 minutes there was a decrease in myocardial blood flow (upward deflection of the temperature record) despite the slightly elevated systemic arterial pressure. This is indicative of coronary vasoconstriction, initiated by the increase in pressure within the lumen of the small intestine. (After Moore and Parratt, 1974.)

considerable physiological and clinical evidence for the concept of reflex coronary spasm as a cause of anginal pain in some patients.

It has been stated above that, for the pharmacologist, there are two main lines of approach to the therapy of angina. The first is a reappraisal of the haemodynamic changes that occur during angina.

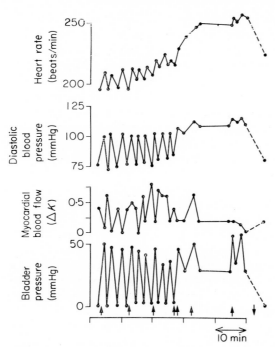

FIG. 2. Evidence for a reflex coronary vasoconstriction elicited by bladder disten-sion in an anaesthetized cat. From above, heart rate (beats per minute), diastolic blood pressure (mmHg), myocardial blood flow (as myocardial thermal conductivity increment, ΔK, c.g.s. units $\times 10^{-4}$) and bladder pressure (mmHg). The bladder volume was increased in stages (indicated by the arrows) and this usually resulted in spontaneous changes in bladder pressure. Each rise in bladder pressure resulted in an increase in diastolic pressure and heart rate but a *decrease* in myocardial blood flow, as measured by a heat clearance technique. (After Moore and Parratt, 1974.)

3   Haemodynamic changes during myocardial ischaemia

One of the most significant advances in angina pectoris arose from studies indicating that angina pectoris results from acute and reversible left ventricular failure. These haemodynamic changes have been well sum-marized by Parker (Parker, 1972a; 1972b) and by Ross (1971). During exercise there is an abnormal elevation of pulmonary arterial and wedge pressures (Müller and Rørvik, 1958) and of left ventricular end-diastolic pressure (Ross *et al.*, 1962; Parker *et al.*, 1966; Wiener *et al.*, 1968; Sharma and Taylor, 1970; Lichtlen, 1970). Left ventricular end-diastolic pressures (LVEDP) as high as 30–40 mmHg have been re-corded during angina precipitated by exercise; the normal range during exercise is 8–10 mmHg. This abnormal elevation of LVEDP during exertional angina is accompanied by a subnormal increase in stroke output and work (Sharma and Taylor, 1970; Parker, 1972a; 1972b). This means that left ventricular function curves (the Frank-Starling relationship relating stroke work to left ventricular filling pressure) are displaced downwards and to the right. A given work load is thus only achieved at abnormally high filling pressures. These changes are indicative of depressed left ventricular function and are accompanied by pain, breathlessness and by characteristic electrocardiographic ST segment changes. There are two possible explanations for the increased LVEDP during exercise-induced angina. Firstly, it may result from an increased diastolic volume, subsequent to depressed myocardial contractility and cardiac dilatation. There is some evidence that this occurs in at least some anginal patients (Dwyer, 1970). A second, and more likely, explanation is a decreased ventricular compliance (or "give", $\Delta V / \Delta P$). This increase in wall "stiffness" may be due to myocardial fibrosis. These cardiac changes may be accentuated by venous constriction induced by increased circulating levels of catecholamines. There is some interesting recent evidence (Robinson, 1974) suggesting that the veins of patients with angina may be more sensitive to the constrictor action of catecholamines than those of normal individuals.

There are two important consequences of the abnormal elevation in LVEDP and of depressed myocardial function. Firstly, the increased stretch of the myocardial fibres increases myocardial wall tension (or stress). This is determined by ventricular pressure, wall thickness and intraventricular volume, and can be calculated from the Laplace relationship for a spheroid chamber ($T = Pr/2h$, where T = tension, P = pressure, r = the radius and h = wall thickness). Since tension in the myocardial wall is a most important determinant of myocardial oxygen consumption (Sonnenblick et al., 1968; Braunwald, 1971) "the onset of acute left ventricular failure will in itself result in a further increase in myocardial oxygen consumption" (Sharma and Taylor, 1970).

The second consequence of the abnormal elevation in LVEDP is a reduction in blood flow to the deep (endocardial) layers of the ventricular wall (Moir and De Bra, 1967; Becker and Pitt, 1971). Blood flow to the endocardium takes place predominantly during diastole since this is the only period during the normal cardiac cycle when pressure in the perfusing artery exceeds the intramyocardial pressure surrounding the deep endocardial vessels. During systole the pressure, both within the lumen of the left ventricle and within the inner region of the myocardial muscle mass, exceeds the pressure in the coronary artery (Kirk and Honig, 1964a; Brandi and McGregor, 1969; Armour and Randall, 1971; Baird et al., 1970). Significant blood flow during systole is only possible to the outer (epicardial) regions where intramyocardial systolic pressures are considerably below those attained in the deeper regions (Armour and Randall, 1971). Assuming that the diastolic intramyocardial pressure surrounding the small blood vessels of the endocardium approximates to the diastolic pressure in the lumen of the ventricle (a not unreasonable assumption, Baird et al., 1970) then the normal diastolic perfusion pressure for the endocardium would be diastolic coronary artery pressure (about 80 mmHg) minus LVEDP (which is about 5–10 mmHg), i.e. about 70 mmHg. This is drastically reduced when the lumen of the coronary artery is restricted (Perlroth and Harrison, 1969) and, of course particularly, when the artery is completely occluded. For example, following acute coronary artery ligation in dogs, the diastolic pressure distal to the point of ligation is of the order of 20–30 mmHg, depending upon the degree of the collateral circulation (Schaper, 1971; Marshall et al., 1974). Since, under these conditions of acute myocardial ischaemia, there is also depression of left ventricular function and an elevated diastolic pressure within the lumen of the ventricle (and therefore presumably around the endocardial vessels) there is only a very small, and quite inadequate, perfusion pressure for the subendocardium. This perfusion pressure has been termed the "subendocardial driving pressure", SEDP, by Marshall and Parratt (1973b; 1974b) and its calculation is illustrated in Fig. 3. Blood flow to the endocardium, under conditions of myocardial ischaemia, will thus depend upon: (a) subendocardial driving pressure; and (b) the duration of diastole (the "effective perfusion period") (Fig. 3; see also Buckberg et al., 1972; Neill et al., 1973).

Under the haemodynamic conditions present in the anginal patient under stress there is therefore a disproportionate reduction in subendocardial blood flow and this is almost certainly responsible for the greater susceptibility to myocardial cellular injury of this region (Jennings, 1969; Jennings et al., 1969; Jennings and Ganote, 1972).

We are now in a position to summarize the essential haemodynamic changes which occur during exertion in the anginal patient (Fig. 4). The increased myocardial oxygen demands are not matched by a proportionate increase in myocardial blood flow because of a restriction to flow (atherosclerosis or vasospasm) in the coronary arteries. There is underperfusion of the endocardial cells with subsequent anaerobic metabolism (indicated by a rise in the lactate to pyruvate ratio—Bassenge et al., 1970), acute left ventricular failure, a reduction in stroke volume, an elevation in left ventricular filling pressure and a subsequent increase in intramyocardial wall tension. This increase in wall tension (and possible increase in cardiac dimensions) will further increase both myocardial oxygen de-

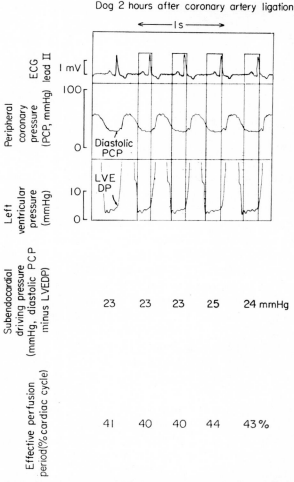

FIG. 3. The calculation of subendocardial driving pressure and effective (diastolic) perfusion time. The dog was anaesthetized with trichlorethylene and the left anterior descending coronary artery ligated 2 h prior to the above record being taken. From above, the electrocardiogram (lead II), the pressure in the stump of the ligated coronary artery (peripheral coronary pressure, mmHg), and left ventricular pressure recorded at high gain to allow the accurate measurement of LVEDP. Subendocardial driving pressure is the difference between the pressure in the ligated coronary artery and the pressure within the lumen of the left ventricle during diastole (which is the only period when perfusion of the subendocardium can occur).

mands and, because of the mechanical pressure on the vessels, the resistance to flow in the deeper regions of the left ventricular wall. These

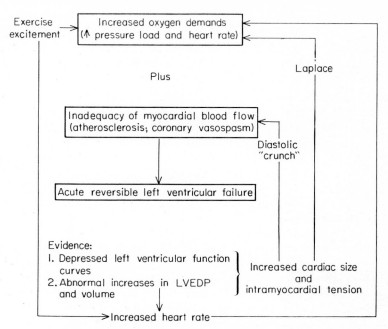

FIG. 4. Haemodynamic changes during the anginal syndrome.

haemodynamic changes are readily reversed when exercise is terminated, the reasons being the abrupt reduction in cardiac work (and therefore myocardial oxygen demands) and the fact that motionless standing leads to the pooling of blood in the lower extremities and hence decreases venous return.

These haemodynamic changes suggest at least three pharmacological approaches to the problem of angina. The vicious circle outlined in Fig. 4 could be interrupted: (i) by decreasing myocardial oxygen demands; (ii) by improving myocardial performance; (iii) by decreasing left ventricular filling pressure. These can be achieved by the use of β-adrenoceptor blocking agents, cardiac stimulants and nitroglycerin respectively.

4   Pharmacological approaches to anginal therapy arising from a consideration of haemodynamic changes

4.1   REDUCTION IN MYOCARDIAL OXYGEN DEMANDS: β-ADRENOCEPTOR BLOCKING AGENTS

The dominant influence on the frequency and severity of angina is increased activity of the sympathetic nervous system leading to a release of noradrenaline. This increased activity may result from emotional stress (e.g. excitement, anger, the tension associated with a change in occupation or with the remembrance of an emotionally charged event), with increased muscular effort (walking up an incline, lifting, exercise after meals) or with exposure to cold. Noradrenaline may also be released after occlusion or obstruction of a coronary artery. Increased plasma and urinary noradrenaline levels have been found during angina (Gazes *et al.*, 1959; Miyahara, 1969), following myocardial infarction (Valori *et al.*, 1967a; 1967b; Hayashi *et al.*, 1969) and after the occlusion of a major branch of the left coronary artery in experimental animals (Lammerant *et al.*, 1966; Staszewska-Barczak and Ceremuzynski, 1968; Shahab *et al.*, 1969).

Released catecholamines would be expected to increase heart rate, the velocity of shortening of cardiac muscle fibres and arterial blood pressure. These haemodynamic changes would result in an increase in myocardial oxygen consumption and there is some evidence that this may be out of proportion to the haemodynamic changes. Thus Raab has argued that the increased cardiac oxygen consumption is excessive and "wasteful" because, under the influence of catecholamines, a reduced fraction of oxidative energy is translated into useful mechanical energy (Raab, 1962). This is the so-called "oxygen wasting" effect of catecholamines (Fawaz and Tutunji, 1960). The increase that occurs in myocardial metabolic heat production after catecholamine administration (Parratt, 1969b; 1969c) also cannot be explained solely by changes in muscle length or tension. In isolated cardiac muscle adrenaline increases not only "additional heat" (the heat liberated when a muscle either shortens or develops tension) but also the tension (or muscle length) independent component (Gibbs, 1967; Gibbs *et al.*, 1967). β-Adrenoceptor blocking agents antagonize catecholamine-induced increases in myocardial oxygen consumption and also in metabolic heat production (Parratt, 1969b; Parratt and Wadsworth, 1970). The most likely explanation for the efficacy of β-adrenoceptor blocking agents in angina is the resultant reduction in myocardial oxygen demand (Shanks, 1967). The rationale for their use in conditions, such as angina, where there is an imbalance between myocardial oxygen supply and demand, was well summarized by Professor J. W. Black, who was responsible for developing this research programme at the Pharmaceutical Division of Imperial Chemical Industries. "We hoped that beta-adrenergic blockade would reduce the consumption of oxygen by the ischaemic myocardium and thus have the same net effect as increasing its oxygen supply. The possibility that the treatment of patients with myocardial ischaemia with adrenergic beta-receptor antagonists might prolong their lives was part of our speculations about the therapeutic use of these drugs" (Black, 1967). Although there is little doubt about the usefulness of such agents in angina there is, as yet, no evidence that they actually prolong the life of such patients. The basic concept that β-adrenoceptor blocking agents are beneficial to the patient with angina because they decrease myocardial oxygen demand has already been comprehensively discussed (for example by Charlier, 1971, and by Fitzgerald, 1972). However, more recent experimental and clinical work suggests there may be other explanations for their efficacy and this is now summarized.

4.1.1 β-Adrenoceptor blocking agents and the extent of myocardial ischaemic injury

In dogs, following occlusion of a major branch of the left coronary artery, propranolol (Maroko et al., 1971; Maroko et al., 1972) and practolol (Libby et al., 1973) reduce the extent and severity of myocardial ischaemic injury as assessed by a reduction in ST segment elevation and by myocardial creatine phosphokinase estimations. There is also some earlier evidence, again in anaesthetized dogs, that, when administered before coronary artery occlusion, propranolol reduces the degree of the resulting myocardial infarction (Grayson et al., 1968). In patients with acute myocardial infarction both of these β-adrenoceptor blocking agents again reduce both the area, and mean height, of ST segment elevation as assessed by multi-electrode praecordial electrocardiograms (Pelides et al., 1972; Maroko et al., 1972). This decrease in the severity of myocardial injury has been attributed to a reduction in myocardial oxygen consumption (Maroko et al., 1971) although the results of the Hammersmith group (Pelides et al., 1972) indicate that there is in fact no correlation between the change in the area, or degree, of ST segment elevation and the change in heart rate. Other haemodynamic parameters, which would influence myocardial oxygen consumption (such as left ventricular dP/dt max, LVEDP and systemic arterial pressure) were not influenced by practolol in a dose that markedly decreased ST segment elevation. The absence of changes in blood flow and in oxygen availability, extraction and consumption in the ischaemic area after the administration of practolol to anaesthetized dogs is illustrated in Table 1 (Marshall and Parratt, 1974c). This is in marked contrast to what happened in the apparently normal surrounding myocardium, where practolol decreased blood flow and oxygen consumption (Table 1) without changing the ratio of myocardial oxygen consumption to oxygen availability. The only significant change that occurred in the ischaemic area in these experiments was a decrease in intramyocardial temperature; this also

TABLE 1

Effects of practolol (0.5 mg kg^{-1}) on myocardial blood flow and oxygen handling in anaesthetized dogs 2 h after acute coronary artery ligation (mean $\pm$ S.E. of mean) (from Marshall and Parratt, 1974c)

Blood flow	Normal myocardium		Acutely ischaemic myocardium	
	Before practolol	After practolol	Before practolol	After practolol
(ml min^{-1})^a	134 ± 20	102 ± 21^b	28 ± 6	28 ± 5
Myocardial oxygen availability (ml min^{-1})^a	42 ± 7	32 ± 7^b	8 ± 2	8 ± 1
Coronary sinus or venous P_{O_2} (mmHg)	33 ± 3	30 ± 2	34 ± 3	32 ± 2
Myocardial oxygen consumption (ml min^{-1})^a	24 ± 4	15 ± 2^b	4.9 ± 1.1	4.6 ± 0.8
Myocardial oxygen extraction (%)	54 ± 5	57 ± 4	56 ± 4	57 ± 4

This dose of practolol decreased heart rate (from 198 ± 13 to 151 ± 17 beats min^{-1}), cardiac output (from 2.0 ± 0.3 to 1.2 ± 0.2 l min^{-1}) and subendocardial driving pressure (from $+5$ mmHg to -4 mmHg). The decrease in driving pressure would be offset by the increase in diastolic filling time resulting from the bradycardia.

^{a} For the ischaemic myocardium the values quoted are as ml 100 g^{-1} min^{-1}.

^{b} $P < 0.01$.

occurred, and to a greater extent, in the adjacent "normal" regions. Although the results outlined in Table 1 indicate that practolol reduces ST segment elevation without changing blood flow or oxygen consumption in the ischaemic area, they do not exclude the possibility that some redistribution of blood flow has occurred. In normal anaesthetized dogs

$$ArOCH_2\underset{\underset{\text{OH}}{|}}{C}HCH_2NHCH(CH_3)_2$$

Propranolol: Ar=

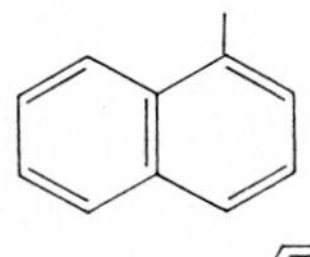

Practolol: Ar=CH$_3$CONH

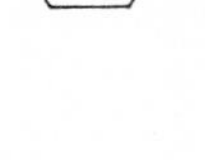

radioactive microspheres of 15 μm diameter are fairly evenly distributed between the deeper (endocardial) and superficial (epicardial) regions of the ventricular wall, with a ratio of flow to the endocardium to flow to the epicardium between 0·99 and 1·2 (Fortuin *et al.*, 1971; Becker *et al.*, 1971). The subendocardium is thus believed to be adequately perfused (see Moir, 1972). The administration of propranolol, although it is known to decrease total myocardial blood flow (Parratt and Grayson, 1966; Parratt, 1969b), nevertheless *increased* the ratio of endocardial to epicardial blood flow (Moir and De Bra, 1967; Fortuin *et al.*, 1971) and usually increased endocardial Po_2 (Moss *et al.*, 1970; Winbury *et al.*, 1971b). Perfusion of the deeper regions of the left ventricular wall is thus favoured. Similar results have been obtained in the acutely ischaemic myocardium, for example after the occlusion of a branch of the left coronary artery. A severe reduction in coronary perfusion pressure, such as occurs after acute coronary artery occlusion, results, as we have indicated above, in a marked, and disproportionate, subendocardial underperfusion. After the administration of propranolol ($1·0$ mg kg^{-1}) Becker and his colleagues (Becker *et al.*, 1971) observed an increase in the LV_{endo}/LV_{epi} ratio (I/O) in both normal and ischaemic regions. The most likely explanations for this increase in endocardial perfusion after β-adrenoceptor blockade are the increased diastolic time (since diastole is the period when endocardial perfusion occurs) and the reduced intramyocardial systolic pressure, allowing blood flow to the subendocardium during systole. Subendocardial driving pressure during diastole is in fact slightly reduced (Table 1).

4.2   IMPROVEMENT OF MYOCARDIAL PERFORMANCE

4.2.1   *Cardiac glycosides*

If, as indicated above, angina pectoris is a form of acute, but reversible, left ventricular failure, then the use of a drug that improves ventricular performance would appear to be indicated. Digitalis glycosides have been used in angina with conflicting results (Malmborg, 1965; Glancy *et al.*, 1971; Aronow, 1973). By increasing the force of contraction they would increase myocardial oxygen consumption. This would, however, be offset by reductions in LVEDP and volume and therefore in wall tension and in cardiac size, factors which would reduce oxygen demand. The most recent study (Harding *et al.*, 1973) concluded that digoxin is worth a trial in the treatment of nocturnal angina, one cause of which is the shift of fluid from the systemic to the pulmonary circulation that occurs in the recumbent position and which may precipitate congestive heart failure.

4.2.2   *Oxyfedrine*

A rather different approach to the use of cardiac stimulants in the alleviation of anginal symptoms has been the recent use of oxyfedrine. There is some evidence from double-blind trials (for references see Parratt, 1974) indicating that oxyfedrine is an effective antianginal drug. It is a partial agonist at β-adrenoceptors, that is, it exerts sympathomimetic effects on atria, and on a variety of smooth muscle preparations, in similar concentrations to those which antagonize the effects of β-adrenoceptor stimulants such as isoprenaline. Oxyfedrine substantially decreases LVEDP and end-diastolic volume, heart size and metabolic heat production in anaesthetized cats (Moore and Parratt, 1972). The result is a reduction in wall tension, which is a major determinant of myocardial oxygen consumption (Sonnenblick *et al.*, 1968). In addition, a substantial degree of β-adrenoceptor blockade is obtained on prolonged oral administration

Oxyfedrine

without a reduction either in cardiac output or in left ventricular dP/dt max. (Parratt, 1974). A combination of these haemodynamic effects would adequately explain any antianginal action of oxyfedrine.

4.3   A REDUCTION IN LEFT VENTRICULAR FILLING PRESSURE

This has been suggested as the primary mechanism of action of nitroglycerin in angina and is discussed in detail below (section 5.6).

5   Pharmacology of nitroglycerin – new facts about an old drug

Another pharmacological approach to the therapy of angina pectoris stems from recent work on the pharmacology of nitroglycerin. Although there is some evidence to the contrary (see Aronow, 1972), most physicians would agree that this drug is effective in the treatment of angina. Although it is nearly a century since Murrell (1879) first advocated its use, the precise mechanism of action of the drug is still uncertain. Some of the possible mechanisms are outlined below.

5.1 AN INCREASE IN CORONARY FLOW

This was, until fairly recently, the classical explanation for the anti-anginal action of nitroglycerin. The change in the emphasis on this particular action of nitroglycerin is clearly apparent if one compares Charlier's two reviews on antianginal agents (Charlier, 1961; 1971). In the earlier book Charlier is clearly of the opinion that this is the primary mechanism of action of nitroglycerin; in the second, there is a much greater emphasis on the efficacy of nitroglycerin being due to a reduction in cardiac work (Charlier, 1971, p. 131).

In anaesthetized dogs, with apparently normal coronary arteries, most recent studies confirm that nitroglycerin, injected either intravenously or directly into a branch of the left coronary artery, increases myocardial blood flow, at least transiently (Marchetti et al., 1964; Bernstein et al., 1966; Ross and Jorgensen, 1968; Malindzak et al., 1970; Vyden et al., 1970). In conscious dogs, intravenous and sublingual nitroglycerin causes a coronary vasodilatation which has two distinct components (Vatner et al., 1972): a direct vasodilator effect on the coronary vessels, and a more sustained secondary vasodilatation resulting from a reflex increase in myocardial contractility and heart rate. The reports dealing with the effect of sublingual nitroglycerin in man are more conflicting. It can increase (Bernstein et al., 1966; Cowan et al., 1969) or leave unaffected (Knoebel et al., 1968) myocardial blood flow in normal human subjects; in patients with coronary artery disease myocardial blood flow is decreased after sublingual nitroglycerin in some studies (Gorlin et al., 1959; Bernstein et al., 1966) and increased in others (Cowan et al., 1969). The variability in the response to nitroglycerin in man, and the fact that the changes that do occur are transient and generally unimpressive, suggest that an increase in coronary blood flow is probably not the main reason for the antianginal effect of the drug.

More impressive are those studies suggesting that, while not necessarily increasing *total* coronary blood flow, nitroglycerin may preferentially increase blood flow through the myocardial nutritional circulation, that is, the capillary circulation which permits exchange between blood and tissues. Pathways (such as arterio-venous shunts and non-functioning or "thoroughfare" capillary channels) which do not allow significant exchange to the myocardial cells are referred to as "non-nutritional". Drugs can have quite different effects on these different components of the microcirculation (see Mellander and Johansson, 1968). The view put forward by Winbury (1967; 1971), mainly on the basis of changes in the myocardial clearance of Rb^{86}, is that nitroglycerin increases the "efficiency" of the myocardial nutritional circulation by the combination of a dilatation of large coronary vessels (see also section 5.2.1) and a relaxation of the precapillary sphincters (see also Provenza and Scherlis, 1959). It is fair to add that Winbury's finding that nitroglycerin increases the myocardial clearance of Rb^{86} has not been confirmed by other workers (Somani et al., 1969).

5.2 A REDISTRIBUTION OF CORONARY BLOOD FLOW

Most recent studies using diffusible radioactive indicators (Love and Burch, 1957; Cutarelli and Levi, 1963; Moir and De Bra, 1967; Griggs and Nakamura, 1968; Mathes and Rival, 1971) or labelled microspheres (Domenech et al., 1969; Becker et al., 1971; Fortuin et al., 1971; Becker et al., 1973; Nakamura et al., 1973) have shown that there is an even distribution of blood flow across the left ventricular wall and that the inner (endocardial) layers are adequately perfused. The ratio of blood flow in the inner region to that in the outer (epicardial) layers (i.e. LV_{endo}/LV_{epi} or I/O) is usually not significantly different from unity. Because of the greater intramyocardial pressure and tension in the endocardium (Kirk and Honig, 1964a) there are increased oxygen demands and significantly lower oxygen tensions have been recorded from these deeper endocardial regions (Kirk and Honig, 1964b; Moss, 1968; Winbury, 1971; Winbury et al., 1972). Using large platinum oxygen electrodes values of 26 mmHg for epicardial—Po_2, and 17 mmHg for endocardial, Po_2 appear to be normal in anaesthetized, open-chest, dogs breathing room air (Winbury et al., 1971a). The ratio of blood flow (oxygen supply) to oxygen consumption is therefore higher in the endocardial than in the epicardial regions of the left ventricular wall. Acute myocardial ischaemia (produced by reducing coronary artery perfusion pressure or by complete occlusion of the coronary vessel) results in a disproportionate reduction in endocardial blood flow (Moir and De Bra, 1967; Griggs and Nakamura, 1968; Becker et al., 1971; Becker et al., 1973; Nakamura et al., 1973) and in endocardial Po_2 (Winbury et al., 1971a). This is also a rise in the lactate to pyruvate ratio in the inner layers (Bassenge et al., 1970). The LV_{endo}/LV_{epi} flow ratio can fall from around unity to values around 0·25 to 0·50 (Becker et al., 1973) and is critically dependent upon the pressure in the perfusing coronary artery (Nakamura et al., 1973). Some studies using radioactive labelled microspheres have shown that nitroglycerin (administered intravenously) increases the LV_{endo}/LV_{epi} blood flow ratio both in the normal myocardium (Becker et al., 1971) and in the acutely ischaemic myocardium (Becker et al., 1971; Mathes and Rival, 1971; Nakamura et al., 1973). Although there are isolated studies (by the same authors, Fortuin et al., 1971) indicating that nitroglycerin either does not change the I/O flow ratio, or decreases it by a "steal" of blood flow from deep to superficial myocardial layers (Forman *et al.*, 1973), most of the present evidence favours a nitroglycerin-induced redistribution of blood flow from the epicardium to the endocardium without an alteration in *total* myocardial blood flow. This redistribution of flow would explain the observation of Winbury and his co-workers (Winbury *et al.*, 1971a; Weiss and Winbury, 1972) that nitroglycerin increases endocardial Po_2 whilst reducing (or leaving unchanged) epicardial Po_2. This increase in endocardial Po_2 is most pronounced 4 to 7 minutes after nitroglycerin administration.

The bulk of the evidence at present thus indicates that nitroglycerin redistributes flow within both normal and ischaemic areas of the left ventricular wall by increasing endocardial perfusion and Po_2. An earlier hypothesis that the drug shifts blood from non-ischaemic to ischaemic areas (Fam and McGregor, 1964) has not been substantiated by microsphere studies (Becker *et al.*, 1971). There are three possible explanations for nitroglycerin-induced increases in endocardial blood flow.

5.2.1   *A preferential dilatation of large coronary vessels*

These would be either: (*a*) The large intramural vessels connecting the main coronary arteries with the subendocardial plexus. These vessels penetrate in a perpendicular manner through the myocardium from the superficial epicardial coronary arteries (Fulton, 1965). Or (*b*) the vessels which, under conditions of chronic myocardial ischaemia, give rise to collaterals. There is some doubt as to whether collateral vessels themselves (at least in the early stages of development) are more than passive conducting channels (Schaper, 1971).

The view that the site of the dilator action of nitroglycerin is principally on the large conducting channels rather than on the main resistance segment of the coronary vascular network (the arterioles) has been developed by Fam and McGregor (1968) and by Winbury and his collaborators (1969). It is based primarily on the different effects of nitroglycerin and of those dilator drugs which act at predominantly arteriolar level, such as dipyridamole. Under conditions of chronic myocardial ischaemia nitroglycerin produces a dilatation of large coronary vessels (Fam and McGregor, 1968; Winbury *et al.*, 1969), increases retrograde blood flow distal to a coronary occlusion and increases the oxygen tension within an ischaemic area. In contrast, dipyridamole fails to increase retrograde flow or the Po_2 of the ischaemic region. These results are similar to those obtained in the acutely ischaemic myocardium by Marshall and Parratt (1973a) with vasodilators such as dipyridamole, dilazep (Marshall and Parratt, 1974a) and carbochromene (Parratt *et al.*, 1973) and are interpreted as indicating that vasodilator drugs acting at arteriolar level "steal" blood from ischaemic into non-ischaemic regions.

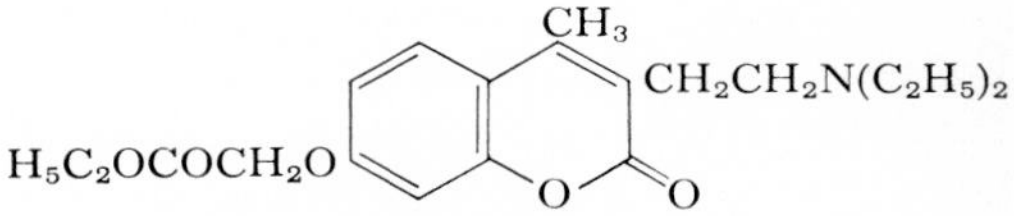

$H_5C_2OCOCH_2O$ — Carbochromene — CH_3 / $CH_2CH_2N(C_2H_5)_2$

$(HOCH_2CH_2)_2N$ — / $N(CH_2CH_2OH)_2$

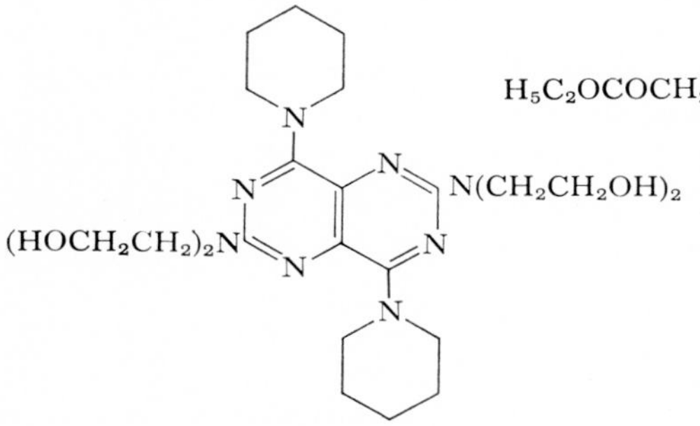

Dipyridamole

CH_3O / CH_3O / CH_3O — $\overset{O}{\overset{\|}{C}}O(CH_2)_3N$ — $N(CH_2)_3O\overset{O}{\overset{\|}{C}}$ — OCH_3 / OCH_3 / OCH_3

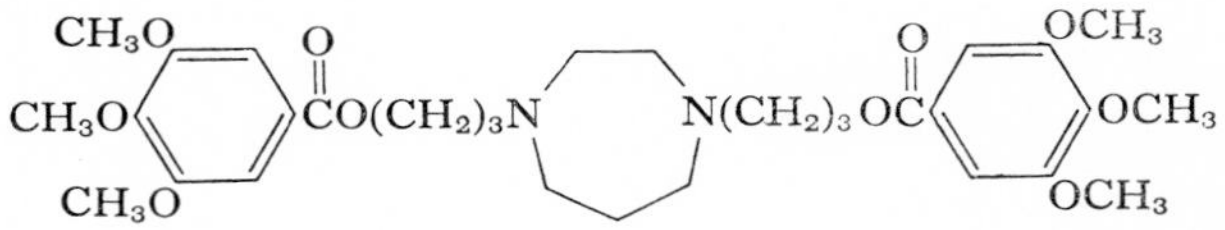

Dilazep

Some support for the concept that nitroglycerin has a preferential dilator action on large coronary vessels has come from work on isolated coronary arteries (Schnaar and Sparks, 1972). Large (2 mm o.d.) and small (0·5 mm) coronary arteries were mounted side by side in an organ bath and contracted with potassium. Nitroglycerin caused a greater relaxation of the larger vessels whereas adenosine caused a greater relaxation of the small vessels. These experiments would tend to support the view that nitrate and non-nitrate vasodilators (such as adenosine, and those drugs that act mainly through an adenosine mechanism, e.g. dipyridamole) have differential effects on the vascular smooth muscle of large and small coronary arteries.

5.2.2 *A reduction in systolic extravascular compression*

Under normal conditions intramyocardial pressure during systole exceeds the pressure in the perfusing coronary artery (Kirk and Honig, 1964a) and blood flow to the endocardium is inhibited. A reduction in peak systolic intramyocardial pressure might allow some blood to flow into the deeper regions of the myocardium during systole. There is some evidence that, under conditions of reduced endocardial blood flow, the administration of nitroglycerin decreases myocardial contractile force in deeper layers of the myocardium, without changing either contractile force in the epicardial regions or systemic haemodynamics (Foreman *et al.*, 1973).

5.2.3   *An increase in the perfusion gradient to the subendocardium*

Blood flow to the endocardium is critically dependent upon the perfusion pressure both in the normal (Buckburg *et al.*, 1972) and ischaemic myocardium (Ledingham *et al.*, 1973; Marshall and Parratt, 1974b). In the acutely ischaemic ventricle the only drugs that improve perfusion are those that increase this trans-ventricular pressure gradient (the subendocardial driving pressure, i.e. the diastolic coronary pressure distal to the point of a coronary occlusion minus the pressure, at this time, within the lumen of the left ventricle—Marshall and Parratt, 1974b). There is good presumptive evidence that nitroglycerin increases subendocardial driving pressure, partly by increasing peripheral pressure in a chronically occluded coronary artery (Schaper *et al.*, 1973) and, more important, partly by decreasing left ventricular and intramyocardial diastolic pressures by a dilator action on peripheral capacitance vessels. This action is discussed in detail in section 5.6.

There is one important piece of evidence that argues against an important primary effect of nitroglycerin on the vessels of the coronary circulation. This stems from a study in which angina was induced, by pacing, in patients with symptomatic coronary artery disease (Ganz and Markus, 1972). Nitroglycerin, administered into the left coronary artery, in a dose (0·075 mg) that markedly increased coronary sinus outflow in normal subjects, failed to reduce the intensity of pain in the patients with coronary artery disease; this was despite the fact that coronary sinus outflow was increased in some of these patients. In contrast, intravenously administered nitroglycerin relieved the angina, the relief of pain being preceded by a fall in arterial blood pressure, in left ventricular end-diastolic pressure—and in coronary sinus outflow. These results were taken by the authors to indicate that "the direct effect of nitroglycerin on the coronary bed plays little, if any, role in the antianginal effect of the drug, which appears to be due entirely to an action on the systemic circulation" (Ganz and Markus, 1972).

5.3   THE CARDIAC STIMULANT EFFECT OF NITROGLYCERIN

Using isolated human and cat papillary muscles (with constant preload and afterload) Strauer and collaborators (Strauer *et al.*, 1971; Strauer, 1973a) have recently demonstrated that, in a concentration range of 0·5 to 1·0 μg ml^{-1}, nitroglycerin increased both developed isometric tension and the maximum velocity of shortening (V_{max}). Force–velocity curves were shifted upwards and to the right in a dose-dependent manner.

Similar results were also obtained with isosorbide dinitrate (Strauer, 1973b) in concentrations 5 to 20 times higher than those of nitroglycerin. A direct positive inotropic effect of nitroglycerin has also been proposed by Raff *et al.* (1970). In a canine preparation, in which aortic blood pressure and left ventricular end-diastolic pressure were held constant, the infusion of nitroglycerin (40 μg kg^{-1} min^{-1}), administered either intravenously or directly into the coronary artery, substantially increased left ventricular dP/dt max (an index of myocardial contractility). Part of this increase in LV dP/dt may have been a consequence of the elevated heart rate but, in view of Strauer's results on isolated cardiac muscle, Lochner's conclusions that "the change in heart rate alone cannot account for the increase in LV dP/dt max" and that "nitroglycerin has a direct positive inotropic effect on the heart", seem reasonable. Under normal (unstabilized) conditions nitroglycerin decreases dP/dt max because of the reduction in arterial pressure and in left ventricular filling pressure.

5.4   CENTRAL INHIBITION OF REFLEX CORONARY VASOCONSTRICTION

This concept is largely the result of the experimental studies of Kaverina and her colleagues at the Moscow Academy of Medical Sciences (Kaverina, 1965; Kaverina *et al.*, 1969). When the central end of a cat tibial nerve is stimulated there is increased electrical activity in efferent sympathetic nerves, a rise in systemic blood pressure and coronary vasoconstriction. These effects were suppressed after the intravenous administration of nitroglycerin (0·5 to 1·0 mg kg^{-1}). Simultaneous with this depression, the noradrenaline content of the medulla oblongata decreased and noradrenaline appeared in the spinal fluid. The depressive effect of nitroglycerin on this vasomotor reflex, which lasted for about 30 minutes, was prevented by the prior administration of reserpine. The conclusion of the Russian workers is basically that nitroglycerin prevents the reflex effects of stimulating afferent A and C fibres by activating free monoamines in structures belonging to the ventro-medial reticular formation. These centres give rise to descending pathways which inhibit spinal vasomotor centres. Although there is some evidence that nitroglycerin depresses noradrenalin-induced increases in blood pressure and myocardial contractile force (Gillis and Melville, 1970) this is unlikely to account for Kaverina's finding since she observed a marked reduction in reflex discharge in sympathetic nerves as well as in the resultant pressor response.

5.5   A DIRECT EFFECT OF NITROGLYCERIN ON CARDIAC MUSCLE METABOLISM

Some of the earlier evidence for a metabolic effect was summarized by

Grayson and collaborators (1967) and by Parratt (1969a; 1969d). The most recent evidence pertinent to this question is that, in myocardial homogenates, nitroglycerin decreases oxygen uptake in a dose-dependent manner (Somani et al., 1969; Levy, 1970). Similarly, measurements of tissue oxygen tension in isolated driven atria have shown that nitroglycerin increases interstitial Po_2 under conditions of constant oxygen supply and cardiac work (Vaghy et al., 1974). The conclusion of the Szeged group (Vaghy et al., 1974), based on these experiments and on two others with mitochondrial preparations, was that nitroglycerin has a direct cardiac metabolic action leading to a more economical use of oxygen and an improved efficiency of oxidative phosphorylation. This action is apparently not shared by other organic nitrates such as isosorbide dinitrate and erythrityl tetranitrate (Levy, 1970).

5.6   PERIPHERAL (VENODILATOR) EFFECT OF NITROGLYCERIN LEADING TO POOLING OF BLOOD WITH SUBSEQUENT REDUCTION IN LVEDP AND VOLUME AND IN MYOCARDIAL OXYGEN CONSUMPTION

We have seen that one of the consequences of exercise in patients liable to angina is a marked, and abnormal, elevation of LVEDP. This is markedly reduced after the administration of nitroglycerin. For example, Parker and his colleagues (see Parker, 1972b) studied the effect of a chewable form of nitroglycerin (in a dose of 0·5 mg) on the response to exercise of patients with coronary artery disease. In those patients with coronary artery disease who developed angina on exercise, the LVEDP rose from a mean of 10 mmHg to a mean of 33 mmHg. The administration of nitroglycerin to these patients reduced the resting LVEDP significantly (from about 8 mmHg to about 4 mmHg) and, after exercise, the LVEDP rose to only 12 mmHg. An earlier study by Lee, Sung and Zaragoza (1970) also clearly demonstrated that nitroglycerin significantly decreased LVEDP and left ventricular end-diastolic volume. Calculations of myocardial wall tension from the law of Laplace showed a reduction of more that 30 per cent. Nitroglycerin has also been shown to reduce ventricular dimensions in man (Williams et al., 1965) and in conscious dogs (O'Rourke et al., 1971). Similar effects of nitroglycerin have also been demonstrated during angina induced by pacing (Chiong et al., 1972). This results in pain, ST segment depression, LVEDP abnormalities and marked myocardial lactate production. After nitroglycerin pain was absent, LVEDP normal, and ST segment depression was less marked. Lactate production did not occur.

The reductions in LVEDP and volume that occur after nitroglycerin appear to be mainly due to a reduction in venous return (Holtermann and

Lochner, 1972). The reduced filling pressure outlasts any reduction in systemic arterial pressure. The effects are in fact strikingly similar to those of a mild phlebotomy (Parker *et al.*, 1970) which reduces LVEDP and has no significant effects on cardiac output, systemic arterial pressure or LV dP/dt. The following evidence supports the hypothesis that the reduction in venous return which follows the administration of nitroglycerin is probably mainly due to dilatation of capacitance vessels.

1. The haemodynamic effects of nitroglycerin, and of nitrites, are a decrease in peripheral vascular resistance and a reduction in stroke volume (Brachfeld *et al.*, 1959; Rowe *et al.*, 1961; Williams *et al.*, 1965). These effects are dissimilar to those induced by vasodilator drugs such as hydrallazine which cause a more pronounced decrease in peripheral resistance and an increased stroke volume.

NHNH$_2$

Hydrallazine

2. Nitrites elicit a pattern of vascular response in skeletal muscle characterized by a pronounced dilatation of postcapillary (venular) resistance vessels and of capacitance vessels and by a moderate dilatation of precapillary resistance vessels (Ablad and Mellander, 1963, in the cat; Ablad and Johnsson, 1963, in man). Precapillary sphincters are not much affected (Johnsson and Oberg, 1968). In contrast, vasodilator drugs like hydrallazine and diazoxide exert their effects predominantly on the precapillary resistance vessels (Ablad and Mellander, 1963; Rubin *et al.*, 1963). This decreases the pre- to post-capillary resistance ratio and favours transcapillary filtration (Ablad and Mellander, 1963). This effect is not seen with the nitrites. Human studies support the evidence derived from animal experiments that the inorganic nitrite ion and the organic nitrites and nitrates exert their main dilator action on capacitance vessels. Thus a reduction in venous tone in the forearm (leading to significant pooling of blood) has been demonstrated after nitroglycerin (Mason and Braunwald, 1965; Williams *et al.*, 1965) and it has been known for many years that sodium nitrite, administered orally, dilates the veins of the hand (Wilkins *et al.*, 1937).

3. Nitroglycerin is much more effective in relaxing isolated venous smooth muscle (contracted with either potassium or noradrenaline) than in relaxing arterial smooth muscle. This is illustrated in Fig. 5. This

"preferential" relaxation of veins is not solely due to the fact that access of the drug to the smooth muscle cells is better in the thinner venous preparation. Some drugs, like papaverine and diazoxide (Fig. 6),

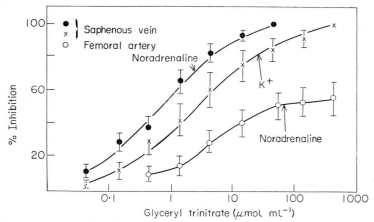

FIG. 5. The effect of glyceryl trinitrate (μmol ml^{-1}) on the response of the isolated dog saphenous vein and femoral artery to noradrenaline and potassium. Significant inhibition of noradrenaline or potassium-induced contraction of the vein was obtained with concentrations of nitroglycerin as low as 1 μmol ml^{-1}. Considerably higher concentrations were required to inhibit the noradrenaline-induced contraction of the isolated femoral artery. The conclusion is that nitroglycerin has a greater selectivity for venous smooth muscle, i.e. for capacitance vessels. (After Mackenzie and Parratt, 1974.)

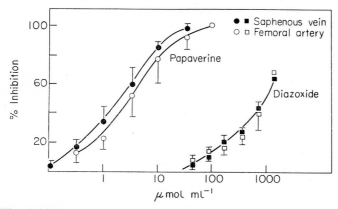

FIG. 6. The inhibition of noradrenaline-induced contractions of dog isolated saphenous vein and femoral artery by papaverine and by diazoxide. In contrast to the effects of glyceryl trinitrate, these two drugs inhibit arterial and venous smooth muscle preparations to the same extent, i.e. they show no particular selectivity for venous smooth muscle. (After Mackenzie and Parratt, 1974.)

inhibit noradrenaline-induced contractions of arterial and venous smooth muscle in similar concentrations, i.e. they show no particular "specificity" for venous smooth muscle. Isoprenaline, like nitroglycerin, has a particular predilection for venous smooth muscle (Fig. 7) and is almost equi-

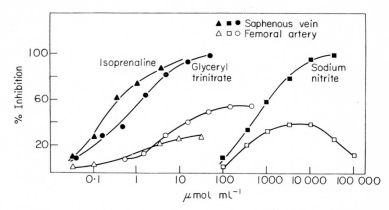

FIG. 7. The inhibition of noradrenaline-induced contractions of dog saphenous vein and femoral artery by isoprenaline, glyceryl trinitrate and by sodium nitrite. Note that all three drugs are more effective on venous smooth muscle than on arterial smooth muscle and that it is never possible to completely inhibit the effect of noradrenaline on the femoral artery. (After Mackenzie and Parratt, 1974.)

potent with nitroglycerin. The mechanism of action is, however, quite different. β-Adrenoceptor blocking agents inhibit the relaxation induced by isoprenaline but have no effect on the relaxation induced by nitroglycerin.

The mechanism through which nitroglycerin relaxes vascular smooth muscle is not well understood. Recent work by Andersson (1973) has shown that the relaxation of smooth muscle that occurs in the presence of nitroglycerin is preceded by an increase in the cyclic AMP content of the muscle. There is a good correlation between the degree of relaxation and the increase in cyclic AMP. Increased cyclic AMP levels may stimulate a Ca^{2+} binding process in smooth muscle and thereby reduce free myoplasmic Ca^{2+} (Andersson, 1972). This may explain the finding that decreasing the calcium concentration of the fluid surrounding isolated vascular smooth muscle increases its sensitivity to nitroglycerin (Lorenzetti et al., 1967).

The above evidence suggests that venodilatation is the main mechanism through which nitroglycerin alleviates anginal pain. By causing peripheral venous pooling it will decrease venous return, ventricular filling pressure and pulmonary artery and capillary pressures. The resultant decreases in cardiac size and wall tension would effectively reduce myocardial oxygen consumption. A reduction in systemic blood pressure (by reducing the resistance to ventricular ejection), and in cardiac output, would result in a decrease in external cardiac work and a further reduction in myocardial oxygen demand. Such a primary action of nitroglycerin on peripheral capacitance vessels would also explain why the direct administration of nitroglycerin into a coronary artery fails to relieve anginal pain. The hypothesis is also not inconsistent with the results (summarized above) indicating that nitroglycerin redistributes blood flow across the wall of the left ventricle in such a way that endocardial perfusion is favoured. By decreasing LVEDP (and presumably also intramyocardial pressure during diastole), as a result of this peripheral action, nitroglycerin would increase the pressure gradient to the inner layers of the myocardium (i.e. the subendocardial driving pressure —Marshall and Parratt, 1974b). Such a "mechanical" decrease in tissue pressure around the blood vessels (the extra-vascular support) would increase the intramural pressure and blood flow (Parratt, 1969a).

The above explanation for the clinical efficacy of nitroglycerin in angina is also supported by recent studies that demonstrate that only drugs that change subendocardial driving pressure, or diastolic perfusion time, are likely to improve perfusion through the acutely ischaemic myocardium (Marshall and Parratt, 1974b). Under these conditions, the myocardial blood vessels are believed to be near-maximally dilated by vasoactive metabolites. A reduction in venous return, and subsequently in cardiac size, is also a possible explanation for the observation of Grayson *et al.* (1967) that, in anaesthetized dogs and rabbits, amyl nitrite markedly reduces myocardial metabolic heat production. Although this could be due to a direct "oxygen sparing" effect of the drug (see section 5.5) a decrease in myocardial metabolic heat production would also result from a reduction in ventricular dimensions and in myocardial wall tension (McDonald, 1971) secondary to the pooling of blood in peripheral capacitance vessels and a decreased venous return.

6 Conclusions: a suggested screening procedure for prospective antianginal agents

Recent studies concerned with the circulatory changes that take place during angina and with the mode of action of nitroglycerin have important consequences for the pharmacologist concerned in predicting the clinical effectiveness of new antianginal drugs. The following is suggested as a screening procedure for prospective antianginal agents and is based on the pharmacology of nitroglycerin. There are already, of course, well laid down principles for screening for prospective β-adrenoceptor blocking drugs.

1. Assessment of venodilator activity on isolated preparations such as the saphenous vein, contracted with potassium or noradrenaline (Fig. 5), or the portal vein of the rat or rabbit. Portal venous preparations have spontaneous myogenic activity and this is reduced in a dose-dependent manner by nitroglycerin (Fig. 8). The effects of drugs on veins should be compared simultaneously with those on arteries (Fig. 7) for some indication of selectivity for capacitance vessels. Another simple, and probably valuable, preparation is the pig coronary artery strip which has been used to examine possible selective dilator effects of drugs on large coronary vessels (Abaitey and Parratt, 1974).

2. Experiments on isolated vascular smooth muscle preparations will, of course, give no indication of drug effects on arteriolar resistance vessels. Although experiments using both saphenous and portal venous preparations would suggest that isoprenaline is an active venodilator (Figs 7 and 8)

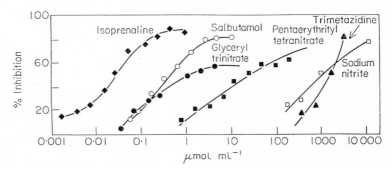

FIG. 8. The inhibition of spontaneous myogenic activity in the isolated rat portal vein by isoprenaline, salbutamol, glyceryl trinitrate, pentaerythrityl tetranitrate, trimetazidine and sodium nitrite. (After Mackenzie and Parratt, 1974.)

it is known that *in vivo* this effect is largely masked by an action on the smooth muscle of the arterioles and that its effect on capacitance vessels is *comparatively* weak (Johnsson and Oberg, 1968). A preparation should therefore be used that will enable the exact site of action of a drug on the microcirculation to be determined. This would be difficult, if not impossible, so far as the myocardial circulation is concerned. An alternative would be to examine the effects on consecutive vascular segments in skeletal muscle. A model that allows an analysis of the effects of drugs on resistance and capacitance vessels, and on the precapillary sphincters, has been described by Mellander (Mellander, 1960; Ablad and Mellander, 1963; Mellander and Johansson,1968) and should yield valuable information about the exact site of action of prospective antianginal drugs on the microcirculation.

3. Ultimately a model should be used that enables the effects of a drug to be examined on oxygen handling (i.e. availability, extraction and consumption) by the acutely ischaemic myocardium. There are two recent examples of such a model. The first is that described by Ledingham, Marshall and Parratt (Parratt *et al.*, 1973; Marshall *et al.*, 1974; Marshall and Parratt, 1974b) and enables the effects of drugs (on blood flow, on oxygen handling and on metabolism) to be examined simultaneously in both normal and acutely ischaemic regions of the canine left ventricular wall. Secondly, there is the model recently described by Szekeres and his co-workers (Csik *et al.*, 1974) in which flow through a branch of the left coronary artery is reduced (by partial constriction of the artery), and the heart paced, until reversible and reproducible ST segment changes occur in the electrocardiogram recorded from epicardial leads. Under such conditions the ratio of myocardial oxygen supply to myocardial oxygen consumption (Szekeres *et al.*, 1967) is decreased, an effect that can be reversed by nitroglycerin.

References

Abaitey, A. K. and Parratt, J. R. (1974). To be published.

Ablad, B. and Johnsson, G. (1963). *Acta Pharmacol. Toxicol.* **20**, 1.

Ablad, B. and Mellander, S. (1963). *Acta Physiol. Scand.* **58**, 319.

Allison, R. B., Rodriguez, F. L. and Higgins, E. A. (1963). *Circulation*, **27**, 170.

Andersson, R. G. G. (1972). *Acta. Physiol. Scand. Suppl.* **382**, 1.

Andersson, R. (1973). *Acta pharmacol. Toxicol.* **32**, 321.

Arbogast, R. and Bourassa, M. G. (1973). *Amer. J. Cardiol.* **32**, 257.

Armour, J. A. and Randall, W. C. (1971). *Amer. J. Physiol.* **220**, 1883.

Aronow, W. S. (1972). *Amer. Heart J.* **83**, 841.

Aronow, W. S. (1973). *Amer. Heart J.* **85**, 132.

Baird, R. J., Manktelow, R. T., Shah, P. A. and Ameli, F. M. (1970). *J. Thorac. Cardiov. Surg.* **59**, 810.

Bassenge, E., Schott, A. and Walter, P. (1970). *In* "Proceedings of the Fifth European Congress of Cardiology" vol. 4, p. 189. Hellenic Society of Cardiology, Athens.

Becker, L. and Pitt, B. (1971). *Ann. Clin. Resl.* **3**, 353.

Becker, L. C., Fortuin, N. J. and Pitt, B. (1971). *Circ. Res.* **28**, 263.

Becker, L. C., Ferreira, R. and Thomas, M. (1973). *Cardiovasc. Res.* **7**, 391.

Bemiller, C. R., Pepine, C. J. and Rogers, A. K. (1973). *Circulation*, **47**, 36.

Bernstein, L., Friesinger, G. C., Lichtlen, P. R. and Ross, R. S. (1966). *Circulation*, **33**, 107.

Black, J. W. (1967). *In* "Drug Responses in Man" (Eds G. Wolstenholme and R. Porter), p. 121. Churchill, London.

Brachfeld, N., Bozer, J. and Gorlin, R. (1959). *Circulation*, **19**, 697.

Brandi, G. and McGregor, M. (1969). *Cardiovasc. Res.* **3**, 472.

Braunwald, E. (1971). *Amer. J. Cardiol.* **27**, 416.

Buckberg, G. D., Fixler, D. E., Archie, J. P. and Hoffmann, J. I. E. (1972). *Circulation Res.* **30**, 67.

Charlier, R. (1961). "Coronary vasodilators". Pergamon, Oxford.

Charlier, R. (1971). "Antianginal Drugs". Springer, Berlin.

Cheng, T. O., Bashour, T., Singh, B. K. and Kelser, G. A. (1972). *Amer. J. Cardiol.* **30**, 680.

Chiong, M. A., West, R. O. and Parker, J. O. (1972). *Circulation*, **45**, 1044.

Christian, N. and Bott, R. E. (1972). *Amer. J. Med. Sci.* **263**, 225.

Cowan, C., Duran, P. V. M., Corsini, G., Goldschlager, N. and Bing, R. J. (1969). *Amer. J. Cardiol.* **24**, 154.

Csik, V., Udvary, E. and Szekeres, L. (1974). *In* "Symposium on Pharmacodynamics of Circulation". (Abstracts), Bratislava, November 1973.

Cutarelli, R. and Levy, M. N. (1963). *Circulation Res.* **12**, 322.

Dimond, E. G. and Benchimol, A. (1963). *Brit. Heart J.* **25**, 389.

Domenech, R. J., Hoffmann, J. I. E., Noble, M. I. M., Saunders, K. B., Henson, J. R. and Subijanto, S. (1969). *Circulation Res.* **25**, 581.

Dwyer, E. M. (1970). *Circulation*, **42**, 1111.

Dwyer, E. M., Wiener, L. and Cox, J. W. (1969). *Amer. J. Cardiol.* **23**, 639.

Eliot, R. S. and Bratt, G. (1969). *Amer. J. Cardiol.* **23**, 633.

Fam, W. M. and McGregor, M. (1964). *Circulation Res.* **15**, 355.

Fam, W. M. and McGregor, M. (1968). *Circulation Res.* **22**, 649.

Fawaz, G. and Tutunji, B. (1960). *Brit. J. Pharmacol. Chemother.* **15**, 389.

Fitzgerald, J. D. (1972). *In* "Effect of Acute Ischaemia on Myocardial Function" (Eds M. F. Oliver, D. G. Julian and K. W. Donald), p. 321. Churchill Livingstone, Edinburgh.

Forman, R., Kirk, E. S., Downey, J. M. and Sonnenblick, E. H. (1973). *J. Clin. Invest.* **52**, 905.

Fortuin, N. J., Kaihara, S., Becker, L. C. and Pitt, B. (1971). *Cardiovasc. Res.* **5**, 331.

Fulton, W. F. M. (1965). "The Coronary Arteries". Thomas, Springfield.

Ganz, W. and Marcus, H. S. (1972). *Circulation*, **46**, 880.

Gazes, P. C., Richardson, J. A. and Woods, E. F. (1959). *Circulation*, **19**, 657.

Gibbs, C. L. (1967). *Aust. J. Exp. Biol. Med. Sci.* **45**, 379.

Gibbs, C. L., Mommaerts, W. F. H. M. and Ricchiuti, N. V. (1967). *J. Physiol.* (*London*), **191**, 25.

Gillis, R. A. and Melville, K. I. (1970). *Eur. J. Pharmacol.* **13**, 15.

Glancy, D. L., Higgs, L. M., O'Brien, K. P. and Epstein, S. E. (1971). *Circulation*, **43**, 45.

Gorlin, R. (1960). *In* "Modern Trends in Cardiology" (Ed. A. M. Jones). Butterworths, London.

Gorlin, R., Brachfeld, N., MacLeod, C. and Bopp, P. (1959). *Circulation*, **19**, 705.

Grayson, J., Irvine, M. and Parratt, J. R. (1967). *Brit. J. Pharmacol. Chemother.* **30**, 488.

Grayson, J., Irvine, M., Parratt, J. R. and Cunningham, J. (1968). *Cardiovasc. Res.* **2**, 54.

Griggs, D. M. and Nakamura, Y. (1968). *Amer. J. Physiol.* **215**, 1082.
Harding, P. R., Aronow, W. S. and Eisenman, J. (1973). *Chest*, **64**, 439.
Hayashi, K. D., Moss, A. J. and Yu P. N. (1969). *Circulation*, **40**, 473.
Hellstrom, H. R. (1973). *Perspect. Biol. Med.* **16**, 427.
Hershberg, P. I. (1971). *Amer. Heart. J.* **81**, 571.
Holtermann, W. and Lochner, W. (1972). *Arzneim. Forsch.* **22**, 1376.
Jennings, R. B. (1969). *Amer. J. Cardiol.* **24**, 753.
Jennings, R. B. and Ganote, C. E. (1972). *In* "Effect of Acute Ischaemia on Myo-
cardial Function" (Eds M. F. Oliver, D. G. Julian and K. W. Donald), p. 50.
Churchill Livingstone, Edinburgh.
Jennings, R. B., Sommers, H. M., Herdson, P. B. and Kaltenbach, J. P. (1969).
Ann. N.Y. Acad. Sci. **156**, 61.
Johnsson, G. and Oberg, B. (1968). *Angiologica*, **5**, 161.
Kaverina, N. V. (1965). "Pharmacology of the Coronary Circulation". Pergamon,
Oxford.
Kaverina, N. V., Bendikov, E. A. and Rosonov, Y. B. (1969). *Pharmacol. Res.
Comm.* **1**, 333.
Kirk, E. S. and Honig, C. R. (1964a). *Amer. J. Physiol.* **207**, 361.
Kirk, E. S. and Honig, C. R. (1964b). *Amer. J. Physiol.* **207**, 661.
Knoebel, S. B., McHenry, P. L., Roberts, D. and Stein, L. (1968). *Circulation*, **37**,
932.
Lammerant, J., Herdt, P. De and Schryver, C. De (1966). *Arch. Int. Pharmacodyn.
Ther.* **163**, 219.
Ledingham, I. McA., Marshall, R. J. and Parratt, J. R. (1973). *Brit. J. Pharmac.* **47**,
626P.
Lee, S. J. K., Sung, Y. K. and Zaragoza, A. J. (1970). *Brit. Heart J.* **32**, 290.
Levy, J. V. (1970). *Brit. J. Pharmacol.* **38**, 743.
Libby, P., Maroko, P. R., Covell, J. W., Malloch, C. I., Ross, J. and Braunwald, E.
(1973). *Cardiovasc. Res.* **7**, 167.
Lichtlen, P. (1970). *Triangle*, **9**, 282.
Lorenzetti, O. J., Tye, A. and Nelson, J. W. (1967). *J. Pharm. Pharmacol.* **19**,
634.
Love, W. D. and Burch, G. E. (1957). *J. Clin. Invest.* **36**, 479.
MacAlpin, R. N., Kattus, A. A. and Alvaro, A. B. (1973). *Circulation*, **47**, 946.
Mackenzie, J. E. and Parratt, J. R. (1974). To be published.
Malindzak, G. S., Green, H. D. and Stagg, P. L. (1970). *J. App. Physiol.* **29**, 17.
Malmborg, R. O. (1965). *Acta Med. Scand.* **177**, Suppl. **426**, 46.
Marchetti, G. V., Merlo, L. and Antognetti, R. M. (1964). *Amer. J. Cardiol.* **13**,
51.
Maroko, P. R., Kjekshus, J. K., Sobel, B. E., Watanabe, T., Covell, J. W., Ross, J.
and Braunwald, E. (1971). *Circulation*, **43**, 67.
Maroko, P. R., Libby, P., Covell, J. W., Sobel, B. E., Ross, J. and Braunwald, E.
(1972). *Amer. J. Cardiol.* **29**, 223.
Marshall, R. J. and Parratt, J. R. (1973a). *Brit. J. Pharmacol. Chemother* **49**, 391.
Marshall, R. J. and Parratt, J. R. (1973b). *Amer. Heart J.* **86**, 653.
Marshall, R. J. and Parratt, J. R. (1974a). *Arch. Pharmacol.* **281**, 427.
Marshall, R. J. and Parratt, J. R. (1974b). *Clin. Exp. Pharmacol. Physiol.* **1**, 99.
Marshall, R. J. and Parratt, J. R. (1974c). *Brit. J. Pharmacol.* In Press.
Marshall, R. J., Parratt, J. R. and Ledingham, I. McA. (1974). *Cardiovasc. Res.* **8**,
204.

Mason, D. T. and Braunwald, E. (1965). *Circulation*, **32**, 755.
Mathes, P. and Rival, J. (1971). *Cardiovasc. Res.* **5**, 54.
McDonald, R. H. (1971). *Amer. J. Physiol.* **220**, 894.
Mellander, S. (1960). *Acta Physiol. Scand.* **50**, Suppl. **176**, 1.
Mellander, S. and Johansson, B. (1968). *Pharmacol. Rev.* **20**, 117.
Miyahara, M. (1969). *Acta Cardiologica*, Suppl. **13**, 174.
Moir, T. W. (1972). *Circulation Res.* **30**, 621.
Moir, T. W. and De Bra, D. W. (1967). *Circulation Res.* **21**, 65.
Moore, G. and Parratt, J. R. (1972). *In* "Action of Oxyfedrine" (Eds E. Gerlach and
  K. Moser), p. 181. Schattauer Verlag, Stuttgart.
Moore, G. and Parratt, J. R. (1974). To be published.
Moss, A. J. (1968). *Cardiovasc. Res.* **3**, 314.
Moss, A. J., Johnson, J. and Sentman, J. (1970). *Cardiovasc. Res.* **4**, 441.
Müller, O. and Rørvik, K. (1958). *Brit. Heart J.* **20**, 302.
Murrell, W. (1879). *Lancet*, **i**, 80.
Nakamura, M., Etoh, Y., Hamanaka, N., Kuroiwa, A., Tomoike, H. and Ishihara,
  Y. (1973). *Cardiovasc. Res.* **7**, 777.
Neill, W. A., Judkins M. P., Dhinsa, D. S., Metcalfe, J., Kassebaum, D. G. and
  Kloster, F. E. (1972). *Amer. J. Cardiol.* **29**, 171.
Neill, W. A., Phelps, N. C., Oxendine, J. M., Mahler, D. J. and Sim, D. N. (1973).
  Amer. J. Cardiol. **32**, 306.
Nigaglioni, A., Finkelstein, D. and Bockus, H. L. (1963). *Amer. J. Cardiol.* **11**,
  253.
Oliva, P. B., Potts, D. E. and Pluss, R. G. (1973). *New Eng. J. Med.* **288**, 745.
O'Rourke, R. A., Bishop, V. S., Kut, P. A. and Fernandez, J. P. (1971). *J. Phar-
  macol. Exp. Ther.* **177**, 426.
Osler, W. (1897). "Lecture on Angina Pectoris and Allied States". Appleton Co.,
  New York.
Parker, J. O. (1972a). *Arch. Int. Med.* **129**, 790.
Parker, J. O. (1972b). *In* "Effect of Acute Ischaemia on Myocardial Function"
  (Eds M. F. Oliver, D. G. Julian and K. W. Donald), p. 288. Churchill Living-
  stone, Edinburgh.
Parker, J. O., Di Giorgi, S. and West, R. O. (1966). *Amer. J. Cardiol.* **17**, 470.
Parker, J. O., Case, P. B., Fareeduddin, K., Ledwich, J. R. and Armstrong, P. W.
  (1970). *Circulation*, **41**, 593.
Parratt, J. R. (1969a). *In* "Progress in Medicinal Chemistry" (Eds G. P. Ellis and
  G. B. West), vol. 6, p. 11. Butterworths, London.
Parratt, J. R. (1969b). *Cardiovasc. Res.* **3**, 306.
Parratt, J. R. (1969c). *In* "Médicaments et Métabolisme du Myocarde" (Eds M.
  Lamarche and R. Royer), p. 217. Nancy.
Parratt, J. R. (1969d). *Acta Cardiol.* Suppl. **13**, 191.
Parratt, J. R. (1974). *Brit. J. Pharmacol. Chemother.* In press.
Parratt, J. R. and Grayson, J. (1966). *Lancet*, **i**, 338.
Parratt, J. R. and Wadsworth, R. M. (1970). *Brit. J. Pharmacol. Chemother.* **38**,
  554.
Parratt, J. R., Ledingham, I. McA. and McArdle, C. S. (1973). *Cardiovasc. Res.* **7**,
  401.
Pelides, L. J., Reid, D. S., Thomas, M. and Shillingford, J. P. (1972). *Cardiovasc.
  Res.* **6**, 295.
Perlroth, M. G. and Harrison, D. C. (1969). *Clin. Pharmacol. Ther.* **10**, 499.

Provenza, V. and Scherlis S. (1959). *Circulation Res.* **7**, 318.
Raab, W. (1962). *Amer. J. Cardiol.* **9**, 576.
Raff, W. K., Drechsel, U., Scholtholt, J. and Lochner, W. (1970). *Pfluegers Arch. Gesamte. Physiol. Menschen Tiere.* **317**, 336.
Robinson, B. F. (1974). To be published. (This symposium).
Ross, R. S. (1971). *Brit. Heart J.* **33**, 173.
Ross, G. and Jorgensen, C. (1968). *Amer. Heart J.* **76**, 74.
Ross, R. S., Schwartz, N., Gaertner, R. A. and Friesinger, G. C. (1962). *J. Clin. Invest.* **41**, 1395.
Rowe, G. G., Chelius, C. J., Afonso, S., Gurtner, H. P. and Crumpton, C. W. (1961). *J. Clin. Invest.* **40**, 1217.
Rubin, A. A., Zitowitz, L. and Hausler, L. (1963). *J. Pharmacol. Exp. Ther.* **140**, 46.
Schaper, W. (1971). "The Collateral Circulation of the Heart". North-Holland, Amsterdam.
Schaper, W., Lewi, P., Flameng, W. and Gijpen, L. (1973). *Basic Res. Cardiol.* **68**, 3.
Schnaar, R. L. and Sparks, H. V. (1972). *Amer. J. Physiol.* **223**, 223.
Shahab, L., Wollenberger, A., Haase, M. and Schiller, U. (1969). *Acta Biol. Med. Ger.* **22**, 135.
Shanks, R. G. (1967). *In* "Problems in Laboratory Evaluation of Antianginal Agents" (Ed. M. M. Winbury), p. 41. North-Holland, Amsterdam.
Sharma, B. and Taylor, S. H. (1970). *Lancet,* **ii**, 902.
Somani, P., Bachand, R. T., Hardman, H. F. and Laddu, A. R. (1969). *Eur. J. Pharmacol.* **8**, 1.
Sonnenblick, E. H., Ross, J. and Braunwald, E. (1968). *Amer. J. Cardiol.* **22**, 328.
Staszewska-Barczak, J. and Ceremuźyński, L. (1968). *Clin. Sci.* **34**, 531.
Strauer, B. E. (1973a). *Z. Kardiol.* **63**, 97.
Strauer, B. E. (1973b). *Int. J. Clin. Pharmacol.* **8**, 30.
Strauer, B. E., Westberg, C. and Tauchert, M. (1971). *Pfluegers Arch. Gesamte. Physiol. Menschen Tiere.* **324**, 124.
Szekeres, L., Papp, J. G. and Fischer, E. (1967). *Eur. J. Pharmacol.* **2**, 1.
Vághy, P., Bor, P., Csete, K. and Szekeres, L. (1974). *In* "Symposium on Pharmacodynamics of Circulation". (Abstracts) Bratislava, November 1973.
Valori, C., Thomas, M. and Shillingford, J. (1967a). *Amer. J. Cardiol.* **20**, 605.
Valori, C., Thomas, M. and Shillingford, J. P. (1967b). *Lancet,* **i**, 127.
Vatner, S. F., Higgins, C. B., Millard, R. W. and Franklin, D. (1972). *J. Clin. Invest.* **51**, 2872.
Vyden, J. K., Carvalho, M., Boszormenyi, E., Lang, T-W., Bernstein, H. and Corday, E. (1970). *Amer. J. Cardiol.* **25**, 53.
Weiss, H. R. and Winbury, M. M. (1972). *Microvasc. Res.* **4**, 273.
Wiener, L., Dwyer, E. M. and Cox, J. W. (1968). *Circulation,* **38**, 240.
Wilkins, R. W., Haynes, F. W. and Weiss, S. (1937). *J. Clin. Invest.* **16**, 85.
Williams, J. F., Glick, G. and Braunwald, E. (1965). *Circulation,* **32**, 767.
Winbury, M. M. (1967). *In* "Problems in Laboratory Evaluation of Antianginal agents" (Ed. M. M. Winbury), p. 26. North-Holland, Amsterdam.
Winbury, M. M. (1971). *Circulation Res.* 28 and 29, Suppl. 1. 140.
Winbury, M. M., Howe, B. B. and Hefner, M. A. (1969). *J. Pharmacol. Exp. Ther.* **168**, 70.
Winbury, M. M., Howe, B. B. and Weiss, H. R. (1971a). *J. Pharmacol. Exp. Ther.* **176**, 184.

Winbury, M. M., Weiss, H. R. and Howe, B. B. (1971b). *Eur. J. Pharmacol.* **16,** 271.
Winbury, M. M., Weiss, H. R. and Howe, B. B. (1972). *In* "Myocardial Blood Flow in Man" (Ed. A. Maseri), p. 37. Minerva Medica, Turin.

Subject Index

Cumulative Index of Authors

Cumulative Index of Titles

DATE DUE
